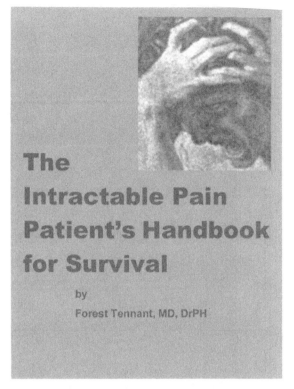

The Intractable Pain Patient's Handbook for Survival

by

Forest Tennant, MD, DrPH

ORIGINAL 2007 COVER FOR THE INTRACTABLE PAIN PATIENT'S HANDBOOK FOR SURVIVAL

The picture of the man with head grasped in his hands is obviously in great agony. This picture was on the original survival handbook written in 2007. I selected this picture not only because it depicts the man's ungodly, indescribable pain, but his fingers reflect that he has been ill for some time and has intractable pain. Note the spindling of his fingers due to tissue deterioration and muscle wasting. His finger joints are enlarged, and his fingers are bent. Overall, he portrays the image of a person who has been in intractable pain for a long time, has malnutrition, and arthritis of his joints either as part of his underlying cause of pain or due to the autoimmunity that may accompany intractable pain.

INTRACTABLE PAIN PATIENT'S HANDBOOK FOR SURVIVAL

By

Forest Tennant

Published by the
Tennant Foundation
West Covina, California

ISBN: 9781955934121
Library of Congress Control Number: 2021916464

Ordering Information:

Special discounts are available on quantity purchases by corporations, associations, educators, and others. For details, contact one of the parties listed below.

U.S. trade bookstores and wholesalers: Please contact
Nancy Kriskovich Tel: (406)249-2002;
or email snkriskovich@gmail.com
Medical Research and Education Project
c/o Nancy Kriskovich
14 Hidden River Lane
Bigfork, MT 59911

All proceeds from the sale of this book will go to the Medical Research and Education Projects sponsored by the
TENNANT FOUNDATION.
336 ½ S. GLENDORA AVENUE
WEST COVINA, CA 91790-3060
A 501(c)(3) Non-profit Organization

ACKNOWLEDGEMENTS

TENNANT FOUNDATION BOARD OF DIRECTORS

Chairperson: Jerry Muszynski
President: Forest Tennant
Vice President: Miriam Tennant
Secretary: Kathy Clark
Treasurer: James Hetzel

BOARD MEMBERS

Doran Barnes
Steve Castillo
Sander De Wildt
Don Scheliga
Vicki Scheliga
Tony Song
Ken Yoho

MEDICAL RESEARCH AND EDUCATION COMMITTEE

Chairperson: Ingrid Hollis
Lynn Ashcraft
Donna Corley
K. Scott Guess, Pharm D
Kristen Ogden
Rhonda Posey
ReAnn S. Rothwell

ACKNOWLEDGMENTS

This book could not have been researched and written without the technical assistance of Becky and Tom Marino and Nancy Kriskovich.

DEDICATION

This handbook is dedicated to the physicians who championed the belief and practiced their trade to ensure that no one lived or died in agonizing pain or had their life shortened due to deprivation of opioids or other critical medication.

Table of Contents

AUTHOR'S INTRODUCTION

In 2007 I wrote the handbook which is published here. It has never been officially published as my original intent was to provide a guide for my own intractable pain (IP) patients. Beginning shortly after I wrote the handbook and started to give it to my patients and families, it began to show up on multiple websites. One site claimed it was downloaded by over 100,000 people. Much to my surprise the handbook hasn't "died." In fact, it is being published here "by popular demand." To summarize, I've been prevailed upon by many patients and families to "leave it as it is", don't update or change it. My response is simple. I wrote the handbook in the first decade of this century with the best medical and heart-felt messages I could muster after treating intractable pain patients for thirty years. While basic treatment of IP is eternal, I have added some sections to the appendix of this handbook that I believe will add prospective and guidance.

I began treating intractable pain in 1975 when I discovered that there are a few people in every community who have this miserable, dreaded condition. It wasn't long after I started, that I began to notice that IP was a "different" kind of pain, and that it didn't respond to the usual treatments in medical practice. Since 1975, I have continued to treat and research IP. My major realization was that there is no substitute for treating and ameliorating the basic, or initial, cause of the pain. My second discovery was that if you can't function mentally and physically, you can't heal. Consequently, the first goal of IP treatment is to bring about "enough pain relief to attain good movement and thinking," so treatment can tackle the underlying disease or disorder that caused the pain in the first place.

In this book I've added a pictorial section of historical descriptions about IP and my involvement which have brought us to the present time. IP is a tragic medical disorder that is controversial and poorly understood. I firmly believe that every person with IP and their family need to educate themselves about the disorder and develop their own self-help care plan along with help from their local physicians and nurse practitioners. New ideas and progress have occurred since I began treating the condition about 50 years ago, and new developments are occurring as this book is being written. To bring some of the new research to bear, I've added an appendix section with some practical guidance for IP patients and their family.

A major discovery is that IP is a constant ("24/7") pain that becomes a syndrome, which causes cardiovascular, endocrine (hormone), and autoimmune complications. I'm hopeful that this book will raise awareness of the syndrome and encourage doctors and communities everywhere to tackle this disorder with specific and heartfelt care. Considerable progress has been made over the last two decades in the treatment of intractable pain. The best progress has been made due to diagnostic and treatment measures that help with the recognition and specific treatment of the underlying "initial" cause of the pain. Some examples are systemic lupus erythematosus, rheumatoid arthritis, pancreatitis, sickle cell disease, interstitial cystitis, diabetes, herpetic neuropathies, and cancer. Today, our major causes of the intractable pain syndrome are adhesive arachnoiditis, genetic connective tissue/collagen disorders commonly called Ehlers-Danlos syndromes, brain injuries, severe neurologic trauma, and advanced osteoarthritis.

A goal of this book is to recognize and credit certain people and institutions that have led to scientific knowledge and the growing movement to recognize and treat IP. This book is dedicated to those physicians who believe and do their best to ensure that no one lives or dies while in the agony of IP, and that no one should have their life shortened because they can't obtain opioids or other critical drugs.

PROLOGUE AND HISTORY OF INTRACTABLE PAIN

The first association of the word "intractable" to "pain" that we can identify was in 1933.[8,9] In that year the Shorter Oxford English Dictionary on Historical Principals defined intractable as "not easily treated or dealt with."[9] It also acknowledges a 1607 reference which states intractable is "resisting treatment or effort." British physicians Hunt and Linnett, in 1960, wrote a seminal article simply entitled, "Intractable Pain."[4] In this article they praised the value of anti-inflammatory agents for the treatment of simple chronic pain conditions, but stated that some chronic pain patients were "intractable, "and required narcotic (opioid) drugs for treatment.

Shortly after this article, British and Irish physicians formed an "Intractable Pain Society" to enhance diagnosis and treatment of the condition.[4] The first use of the term to describe physiologic complications of intractable pain was in 1978 when two Canadian physicians (Glynn and Lloyd) used the term "intractable" in a paper entitled, "Biochemical Changes Associated with Intractable Pain."[2] As reported in the British Medical Journal, they found that these patients had elevated carbon dioxide levels due to impairment of breathing caused by the presence of intractable pain. A Philadelphia neurologist by the name of Shenkin, shortly after a blood test for cortisol was developed, found, in 1964, that cortisol levels were pathologically altered in some chronic pain patients.[6]

These studies were the forerunners of a longer list of studies that have demonstrated that persons with intractable pain have objective physiologic abnormalities that separate them from the simple chronic pain patient.[1,3,5,7,10,11] Beginning in the 1990's, some state legislatures began passing intractable pain laws.

These laws fundamentally defined intractable pain as "incurable by any known means." The intent of these laws was to permit physicians to prescribe opioids without retribution or discipline by their state medical boards and justice departments. These laws were helpful for over two decades in that they enabled opioid prescribing for persons suffering from intractable pain as well as enduring research to help struggling and desperate individuals.[3,4]

These laws, however, have had a tragic outcome. In recent years, some states have essentially ignored these laws by prosecuting physicians who prescribed opioids and restricting the availability of opioids even when prescribed to a needy, legitimate intractable pain patient. Basically, these actions have been taken due to the belief by some parties that opioids, even when prescribed to legitimate pain patients, are now overly associated with abuse, addiction, and overdoses to allow medical use even as a last resort treatment.

The term "intractable" has not been embraced by any professional organization. Early in this century, there was a movement to replace the term "intractable" with "high-impact" or "persistent."[1] These terms have not found any widespread acceptance either, as these labels are more ill-defined than the term "intractable." These terms also trivialize those persons with Intractable Pain Syndrome who should be viewed as having a catastrophic illness.

In summary, the term "intractable" has emerged in that it both signifies an incurable state and implies that a subgroup of severe chronic pain patients exists among the population of chronic pain patients.[10,11] The terms "persistent" or "high-impact" pain, and the concept of chronic pain as a disease has not found general acceptance. All persons who have a painful condition that lasts over about ninety days have continued to be labeled as having "chronic pain." Recent research has clarified the issue so that understanding and diagnostic testing can now identify chronic pain patients who started with "simple" chronic pain but have developed a complex of physiologic abnormalities for which the most appropriate name is the "Intractable Pain Syndrome" as constant pain, per se, causes a multitude of physiologic abnormalities.

Although this book maintains its original intent which was to help individual patients find some relief and recovery, it also champions these two long held beliefs of physicians who, over the centuries, have attempted to care and treat the worst of pain problems. First, no person should have to suffer or die in pain if opioids are the only answer. Second, no life should be shortened due to a lack of opioids or other available medications.

REFERENCES

1. Cousins, MJ. Persistent pain: a disease entity. J Pain Symp Manage 2007;33(2S):S4–S10.
2. Glynn CJ, Lloyd JW. Biochemical changes associated with intractable pain. Br Med J 1978;1:280-281.
3. Gunn J, Hill MM, Bradley M, et al. An analysis of biomarkers in patients with chronic pain. Pain Physician 2020;232:E41-E49.
4. Hunt JH, Linnett MJ. Intractable pain. Brit Med J 1960;(June):1726-1729.
5. May A, Boorsok D, Becerra L. Chronic pain may change the structure of the brain. Pain 2008; 137(1):7–15. 28.
6. Shenkin HA. Effect of pain on diurnal pattern of plasma corticoid levels. Neurology 1964;14:1112-1115.
7. Sindall PJ, Cousins MJ. Persistent pain as a disease entity: implications for clinical management. Anesth Analg 2004;99(2):510-520.
8. The History of the Intractable Pain Society of Great Britain and Ireland. Pain 1980;8:121-122.
9. The Shorter Oxford English Dictionary on Historical Principles, Clarend Press, London, (1933) p1035.
10. Tennant F, Hermann L. Intractable or chronic pain: there is a difference. West J Med 2000;173:306.
11. Tennant F, Hermann L. Using biologic markers to identify legitimate chronic pain. Amer Clin Lab 2002;21(5):14- 18.

INTRACTABLE PAIN PATIENT'S HANDBOOK FOR SURVIVAL

2021
reprint of the
2007 original

1. YOU'RE A RARE BIRD

The biggest problem an intractable pain (IP) patient faces for survival is that a bona fide IP patient is a rarity among chronic pain patients. Chronic pain, by standard medical definition, is a pain that is present over ninety days, and which can be continuous or intermittent. Millions of people have chronic pain. Common arthritis, TMJ, carpal tunnel, bunions, and headaches all qualify. However, true IP, as defined here, is constant, severe, disabling pain, which causes changes in pulse rate, blood pressure, and adrenal hormone production. This form of pain is relatively rare. Control of IP requires the daily use of prescription medication. I estimate that one IP case occurs among about every thousand chronic pain patients.

Due to IP's rarity, almost every doctor, insurance plan, hospital, or family member you encounter will initially assume you are just another, average, chronic pain patient who can get by with the standard first- line treatments such as exercise, positive mental attitude, acupuncture, massage, and non-prescription drugs. To survive, you will constantly have to fight this misconception, and you must educate most of the people you encounter.

IP patients all require a custom-made, one-of-a-kind treatment plan. Most physicians and other medical personnel you encounter may be bewildered and even fearful of your treatment, because they may not have encountered another patient with your pain severity.

2. ACCEPT YOUR PLIGHT

There is nothing more demoralizing and depressing than to have severe pain that never stops. It is OK to ask the question. (Why me, Lord?) This is a natural reaction. You can and will repeatedly try to analyze what you could or should have done to prevent it.

No doubt you will try to blame, or finger point someone or some event as the culprit for your problem. You will hope and pray that you are in some nightmare that will be gone when you awake.

Go ahead and cry as often as you need. You probably have every right and reason to feel sorry for yourself. After all, IP is a sorrowful condition.

However, there are two absolute "musts" for IP patients:

1. Do not let pain make you think you are a bad person or some evil spirit. Take it from me: some of God's very best children have IP.

2. Accept the fact that you have IP. Think of it as a disease that can be controlled and, with a little help from medical science, may even be cured someday.

It sounds so obvious and simple, but the hardest thing an IP patient to do is, down deep in your mind, heart, and soul, stop denying that you have a serious, life-shortening, medical condition that will not go away. You have undoubtedly heard, for example, that alcoholics and addicts are often "in denial" that they have a problem. No question about this. It is human nature to deny that one has a serious, incurable disease. There is also no question that an IP patient may have a greater degree of denial than the alcoholic or addict, because so many people ignorantly tell you "your pain is all in your mind." You must accept your plight, because denial will keep you from embarking upon a path that will effectively control your pain, give your life meaning, and extend your life. Every single day you delay effective pain control will cause your body to literally age and your organs rust away. Too long of a delay may leave you in a permanent demented, vegetative state. Bottom line. For whatever reason and whatever the cause, you have IP. Accept the fact that you have IP so you will not become paralyzed due to this condition, and incapable of attacking your problem and aggressively treating it.

2

3. A NEW ATTITUDE: PAIN IS YOUR ENEMY – NOT YOUR SYMPTOM

Always remember that true IP is relatively rare compared to other forms of pain. This understanding is critical since society bombards you with all kinds of clichés and sayings about pain that not only do not apply to you but may likely prove to be destructive.

The statements, "No pain, no gain" and "When the going gets tough the tough get going," are truly positive and meaningful to the healthy sportsman, soldier, or weekend gardener with a typical, run-of-the-mill injury to his or her back, elbow, or knee. Chances are that the injury, once healed, will make the person even stronger and more competitive. After all, many successful champion athletes "tough out" some pain and win. The difference we are talking here concerns pain and nerve damage that is healable, not IP that is caused by some permanent nerve damage and, in most cases, cannot be healed.

Your IP pain is long-standing, constant, keeps you from sleeping, drives up your pulse rate and blood pressure, and alters your adrenal hormone levels. You must remember that your pain is your enemy. To cause it to worsen or flare for any reason may do further damage to nerves and other body tissues that are already permanently damaged.

Your attitude about pain must change. Increased pain hurts you. When the pain flares, your pulse rate increases, and hormones stored in your adrenal gland flood your system causing further body deterioration, rusting, and aging.

Therefore, you MUST do whatever it takes to suppress your pain and prevent flare-ups. You simply want to keep pain as far away and as controlled as possible. Never try to "work through it" or "tough it out" or believe that character and will-power will solve your problem.

4. DEVELOP A SURVIVOR MENTALITY

Now that you have accepted your condition and you begin to consider pain your enemy, you must develop a positive attitude of hope and survivorship. Why? We no longer consider IP entirely hopeless and incurable. Recent medical research advancement is fast and furious. While I make no guarantees, I now see many IP patients who used to have severe, pain 24/7, but now have some pain free hours or even days. There are new terms you must learn along with the word "intractable." First, you must know about the "cardiac-adrenal-pain syndrome." This is essentially the biologic difference between ordinary chronic pain and IP. The life-shortening, debilitating mechanism by which IP destroys a life is the over-stimulation of the cardiac and adrenal hormone systems in the body. A term of hope is "neurogenesis." This means that nerves can regenerate or regrow. At one point, we did not believe this was possible, but now we know differently. This is the key to the cure or permanent reduction of IP. You must stay healthy and live long enough to benefit from all the new scientific developments that are in the pipeline. Another term is "anabolic therapy." Anabolic means to grow tissue. Some new pain treatments are meant to grow nerves and other tissue. Many are truly hopeful such as hormone treatments and nerve stimulation, to name some current front-runners in the race to cure IP. Your immediate job is to stay alive and functioning. Keep the pain away and maintain your mind, body, and social life while awaiting the advances of research and science.

5. YOUR CLOSE AND LOVED ADVOCATE AND CONFIDANT

To survive, defined here as enough pain control to extend your life span and enhance your quality of life, you must have at least one close and loved advocate and confidant. There are many reasons for this.

As you go through life and try to navigate your way through the rocky waters of our medical system, you will need a close advocate to assist you. Long waits, paperwork, and hostile medical personnel are commonplace for an IP patient. The most practical reason you need an advocate who can vouch for your legitimacy and veracity is to convince doctors, dentists, and hospitals that you do not abuse your medication, and that you truly suffer severe, life-threatening pain.

You must understand that doctors are constantly accosted by drug abusers simply to get drugs. These persons complain about headaches, arthritis, or stomach upset just to get drugs to abuse or sell. Unless you possess medical records and an advocate to vouch for your legitimacy, do not expect any physician, pharmacist, or hospital to believe anything you have to say about your pain. Furthermore, do not expect to be treated with decency and respect.

Unfortunately, every doctor, hospital, and pharmacy has been so besieged with drug abusers that they simply will not even deal with an IP patient without an advocate and records to validate your word. Furthermore, doctors are constantly harassed by insurance company "expert consultants," who plague doctors with inquiries which subtly or not so subtly tell the doctor that his pain patients are not really in pain and do not need pain medication.

In addition to medical providers, you may need an advocate to help deal with the intricacies of your health insurance plan and the various agencies that provide disability or worker's compensation benefits. Who should be your advocate? Ideally your spouse or significant other if you are lucky enough to have one. Many IP patients end up divorced or alone since they cannot or will not expend the time, emotion, or love to maintain a marital relationship. If not a spouse, another close family member such as a parent, sibling, child, in-law, friend, or neighbor will do. Just identify someone in whom you can confide, who cares about you, and can accompany you.

There is another benefit to having one or more close advocates and confidants. It makes you a better person and forces you to become a true friend to someone. It is not easy. Despite your pain and misery, you will have to develop an interest in someone else if they are to have an interest in you. True friendships are like plants and pets. They take frequent watering, pruning, feeding, and petting to thrive. So will your advocate. Sometimes this interaction is difficult when you are in constant pain, but you can learn to dig down into your soul and heart to find some real interest in those special people around you.

Through the years some of the most loving couples (including gays and lesbians) I have met are ones in which one member had IP. I have attributed this to the fact that IP patients who truly accept their plight also figure out, better than any other group of people or patients I have ever known, what really counts in life. Love and a few close friends!

6. MAKE AN INVENTORY OF PAIN TRIGGERS

Now that you know that pain is the enemy, you must make an inventory of physical and mental activities and events that cause your pain to flare or worsen. Even though you are aware of most of these, make sure you periodically review your list of pain flares. Every time you discover something new that causes a flare, write it down. This will help you attack the pain before it rears its ugly head. For starters, turn to the "Inventory of Pain Triggers" at the end of this Handbook and complete it. Share your pain flare triggers with family and advocates. They may be able to help you avoid pain flares. If you have a cat, dog, or other pet, they may actually know when your pain is about to flare. An impending pain flare may provide a subliminal signal to a beloved pet that can tip you off that it is time to take some extra preventive measures. For example, your pet may become more affectionate towards you, as if it knows you are in extreme pain.

7. DON'T BUY THE "MAGIC BULLET" CRAZE

Denial, desperation, and misinformation can all lead to poor pain control and continued deterioration. The worst propaganda being pushed upon all chronic pain patients, including those with and without IP, are the elusive "magic bullet" formulas being advanced by the pharmaceutical and medical device industries, unethical practitioners, and some health plans and government agencies. Just look at the ubiquitous advertisements for pain treatment. They almost all try to sell you on the magic bullet, "one way" method to treat your pain. For example, recall all the many pitches you have heard, for such singular "cures" as acupuncture, stimulators, nerve blocks, lasers, medications, and psychotherapy to name a few. The worst deception these days is the fraudulent pitch that pain can be cured by stopping all medications. As if the control is the cause!!

IP patients must continually remind themselves that they are rare patients. The vast majority of chronic pain patients have pain that responds to rather simple, common forms of pain relief such as massage, chiropractic, and non-opioid drugs. IP pain is different. Only potent pain relief measures are effective.

8. MAKE AN INVENTORY OF PAIN RELIEVERS

You have already done an inventory of what triggers your pain to worsen or flare which is a major building block to controlling your IP.

The second step is to do an inventory of everything you know that helps control your pain or prevents even slight pain flares. Sit right down now and review the "Inventory of Pain Relievers" found at the end of this Handbook. IP patients who successfully control their pain simultaneously practice many different control measures. They do not rely on any single measure.

9. ATTACK IP FROM MANY DIRECTIONS AT THE SAME TIME

You can only control true IP by attacking it from many directions at the same time. There is no question about it, bona fide IP will require a foundation of opioid drugs. However, they only work well, over time, if they are part of a multi-component program. Like a good baseball team, a lot of players in many positions must function simultaneously.

Think of your pain control program as though you are putting together a patchwork quilt. You need lots of patches to create one huge quilt. Your pain control program must have many patches – big and small. Do not throw away or discard anything that helps control your pain even slightly. After all, we want to patch you up as best we can!

Put another way, build a program of blocks or steppingstones. Once we identify one stone or block that works, we do not throw it away – we add to it. There is no question about it, control of IP is difficult because it requires many building blocks. Remember this saying, "If you have a winning horse, keep riding it until it drops or a better one comes along."

10. KNOW YOUR CAUSE OF PAIN BY ITS MEDICAL NAME

Provided here is a Table of the most common causes of IP. You do not need to be an expert on causes, but you must know your cause by its accepted medical name. For example, you cannot have plain "arthritis. You have "joint degeneration." You don't have a "bad back" you have "spine degeneration." When dealing with insurance plans and the medical system, you must state your problem as IP secondary to its cause. For example, "IP secondary to spine degeneration."

TABLE OF COMMON CAUSES

- Spine degeneration
- Neuropathies of leg, arm, and chest wall including...
  - Reflex sympathetic dystrophy (RSD, often referred to as complex regional pain syndrome)
  - Fibromyalgia
  - Abdominal adhesions
- Pelvic neuropathies including vulvodynia and prostatodynia.
- Interstitial cystitis
- Headaches
- Joint degeneration - neck, hip, knee
- Systemic lupus erythematosus

---

11. COMPLICATIONS OF INTRACTABLE PAIN

IP has numerous, severe complications which will shorten your life and incapacitate you unless you take the bold measures required to control IP. Totally untreated IP will cause death within days to weeks once it starts. This occurrence, for example, has been observed following injuries to soldiers who could not obtain morphine or other potent pain relievers. Educate all persons you can about these complications. Why? Our health care system and insurance industry, as a group, want to deny that severe complications of IP exist. To acknowledge that these complications exist means that IP must be considered a serious catastrophic disease that is expensive to treat. The list here includes conditions that are caused or worsened by IP.

TABLE OF COMPLICATIONS

- TACHYCARDIA (high pulse rate)
- HORMONE DEFICIENCIES
  (adrenal, thyroid, ovary, testicle, pituitary)
- HEART ATTACK
- STROKE
- OSTEOPOROSIS
- TOOTH DECAY
- LOSS of LIBIDO
- DEPRESSION
- WEIGHT GAIN
- DIABETES
- HYPERTENSION
- HYPERLIPIDEMIA
- MEMORY LOSS & CONCENTRATION
- INSOMNIA
- MUSCLE WASTING
- FATIGUE
- IMMUNE IMPAIRMENT / INFECTIONS
- WEIGHT LOSS / STARVATION

---

12. CARDIAC-ADRENAL-PAIN SYNDROME

Severe, constant IP causes the mid-brain area known as the hypothalamus to over-activate the pituitary and adrenal glands, which in turn produce excess blood levels of adrenaline, cortisol (the body's natural cortisone), and related chemicals. Excess adrenaline causes the pulse rate and blood pressure to rise, and excess cortisol, overtime, causes loss of bone and teeth, osteoporosis, weight gain, hypertension, diabetes, and immune suppression among other complications. IP patients <u>MUST</u> find out if they have this syndrome, because it causes too many serious complications if it is not controlled. For example, a pulse rate or blood pressure that remains high, over time, may cause any one of several cardiovascular complications including arteriosclerosis, angina, heart attack and stroke. It is the author's belief that most IP patients die prematurely of heart or stroke complications. Due to these complications, IP patients must obtain the pain control they need to keep their pulse rate and blood pressure in check.

13. BLOOD PRESSURE AND PULSE RATE- CRITICAL MEASUREMENTS

Uncontrolled IP drives up the pulse rate to over 84 per minute. Many patients go over 100 per minute when their pain is in a flare or breakthrough episode. Blood pressure may also go up over 130/90mm/Hg. It must remain below this figure.

It is critical to understand that uncontrolled pain produces damage and aging to the body, and pulse and blood pressure let you objectively know if you are in adequate control. You MUST obtain a blood pressure and pulse monitor for at-home use. They are now quite inexpensive and can be obtained at most pharmacies. I recommend you check your pulse and blood pressure daily. You particularly need to check it during a pain flare or breakthrough episode to let you know just how much danger you may be in during a flare. For example, if the flare drives up your pulse rate above 120 per minute, you are at serious risk for a heart attack or stroke. I have observed several IP patients who develop angina (severe heart pain) during pain flares and require nitroglycerine. Use your pulse rate and blood pressure to adjust your medication. Always let your medical practitioners know what your pulse and blood pressure readings are running at home. IP that causes blood pressure to elevate will not respond well to the high blood pressure drugs used for ordinary high blood pressure treatment. Only adequate pain control will lower high blood pressure caused by pain.

14. NECESSITY FOR OPIOID DRUGS

A fundamental fact about opioids is that they are the only medication that will truly control IP. Why? The nervous system has specific pain relief trigger points scientifically known as opioid receptors. Natural pain relief in the body is caused by a group of chemicals known collectively as endorphins which attach and activate these receptors. Since these pain relief sites receive endorphins, they are hence called "receptors." Endorphin is so closely related to morphine that the name endorphin is derived from "end," which is Latin for "in the body" and "orphin" which is the last part of the word morphine.

The God-given poppy plant is the source for most medicinal opioids including opium, morphine, codeine, and hydromorphone, among others. Fundamentally, opioid drugs are natural plant or herbal compounds. Consequently, they are quite safe when taken at proper dosages and prescribed by a knowledgeable physician. No other class of drugs now or in the future will likely relieve pain like opioids since the natural endorphins in the brain and opium poppy plant derivatives are essentially one and the same. They do not cause

12

tissue damage like many other medicinals including alcohol, aspirin, acetaminophen, and anti-inflammatory agents, but they can produce sedation, impairment, overdose, and hormone depletion. Historically, they have been widely used since the Egyptian empire and by advanced societies all over the world who cared about the relief of suffering and pain among their inhabitants.

15. BIAS AGAINST OPIOIDS

IP patients must be aware of the history, bias, safety, and true effectiveness of opioids since many parties in modern society have been and continue to be on a campaign to ban or restrict their use. Every IP patient will have to constantly face an ignorant bias against opioids. Bias and ignorance may be thrown in your face by family, friends, doctors, nurses, government officials, employers, and your health plan. The worst offenders, in my experience, are the mental health industry and the sellers of non-opioid pain treatments. Simply put, parties who have a financial interest in keeping patients in uncontrolled pain continually bad-mouth opioids. Be prepared to educate all comers, and above all, remember that IP requires opioids for control. There is no option.

Why the bias? Opioids work too well and there is no substitute. They give an IP patient a meaningful, extended, quality of life. I now have IP patients who have safely and effectively taken high doses of opioids for over twenty continuous years. Current medical knowledge indicates that IP patients can have a normal lifespan if they have access to a dosage of opioids which effectively controls their pain.

The real motivation behind opioid bias is money. Opioids are expensive treatment for health plans including government plans. When IP is properly treated with opioids, the patient no longer must hang out in emergency rooms or hospitals, undergo surgery, or go whimpering to a mental health clinic for "depression" just to get a little relief. Additionally, you do not have to soak yourself in alcohol, buy heroin from drug dealers, or become the neighborhood pothead. I have heard many a government regulator, health plan bureaucrat, and even some of my fellow doctors proclaim to me that they would like to see all IP patients deprived of opioids. Fortunately, these attitudes and biases are slowly disappearing, but always be aware that they exist.

Please know about the biggest racket and fraud going on in medicine today. Believe it or not, some medical hucksters are claiming that opioids cause pain, and your pain will go away if you just detoxify, stop opioids, or get psychological help!! What utter disregard for science and suffering!

In another section of this Handbook there is a section on support groups and advocacy. Every IP patient should join some support group and band with other patients, families, and advocates who support public access to opioid pain relievers and support physician rights to prescribe opioids. I am only able to write this Handbook because of political pressure exerted in recent years on legislative and government regulatory agencies by groups of IP patients, families, advocates, and doctors. Never take your supply of opioids for granted. They work too well and have too many financial enemies. The life you save may be your own.

16. OPIOID CATEGORIES

FIRST STEP OPIOIDS

When you first start opioids for treatment, you will start with one listed in the "First Step Table." These opioids can be taken as needed, or on a regular basis. This group of opioids have few side effects and create little dependence. Some contain acetaminophen, ibuprofen, aspirin, or other potentiators which are compounds that make the opioid act stronger and last longer.

FIRST STEP OPIOIDS	
OPIOID	**COMMON TRADE NAMES**
Hydrocodone	Vicodin®, Lortab®, Norco®
Propoxyphene	Darvon®, Darvocet®, Darvon-N®
Tramadol	Ultram®
Codeine	Empirin®, Fiorinal®
Dihydrocodeine	Panlor®
Pentazocine	Talwin®
Nalbuphine	Nubain®
Butorphanol	Stadol®

Some patients may require two of the "First Step" opioids which may be a preferable treatment approach to the "Second Step Opioids." First Step opioids are short-acting in that they usually provide pain relief for only about two to four hours.

Before going to Step Two opioids, patients should attempt to control their pain with a Step One opioid coupled with one or more of the ancillary medications and treatments listed in this Handbook. Vigorous attempts should be made to avoid Step Two opioids, since they may produce complications.

STEP TWO OPIOIDS

If Step One opioids fail to adequately control pain, an IP patient will have to resort to Step Two opioids. They are much more potent than Step One opioids. They are usually required if pain is severe and constant—meaning it never goes away during the entire twenty-four-hour day unless the patient is asleep. Patients with the "cardiac-adrenal-syndrome" will usually require Step Two opioids. Unfortunately, these opioids may cause constipation, hormone changes, and weight gain. Patients who must take them must learn and practice measures to minimize complications. Some Step Two opioids are often referred to as long acting since they remain in the blood and control pain for several hours.

STEP TWO OPIOIDS	
OPIOID	**COMMON TRADE NAMES**
Methadone	Methadose®, Dolophine®
Morphine	Kadian®, Avinza®
Oxycodone	OxyContin®
Fentanyl	Duragesic®
Levorphanol	Levodromoran®
Oxymorphone	Opana ER®

Long-acting opioid products, including morphine, methadone, oxycodone, and oxymorphone, are to be taken on a regular, fixed schedule. Depending on the opioid, the time interval will be every six, eight, twelve, or twenty-four hours. IP patients should discipline themselves to take their long-acting opioid on a fixed, regular schedule such as when they first awake, noon, late afternoon, and just before bedtime. They are <u>NOT</u> to be taken as needed, and when patients attempt to take them this way, they soon find that their pain is not well controlled. Many patients will also need to use Step One opioids during pain flares or breakthrough pain.

Some of the above are now produced in very innovative formulations. Fentanyl is a skin patch and the morphine formulations listed in the Table above act like a pump in the intestine providing pain relief for as long as twelve to twenty-four hours.

17. BREAKTHROUGH PAIN

Some Step Two opioids are long-acting and prescribed to suppress pain and possibly prevent pain from even occurring. Unfortunately, they may not totally do the job, and pain will flare or "breakthrough" the barrier of the long-acting opioid. A severe breakthrough or flare episode can disable you and send you to bed or worse- to the emergency room. If your pulse rate or blood pressure rises too high during a breakthrough episode, you may even have a heart attack or stroke that could be fatal. Consequently, most severe IP patients will need to master the use of a long-acting opioid and one or more breakthrough opioids.

BREAKTHROUGH PAIN	
OPIOID	COMMON TRADE NAMES
Fentanyl Transmucosal ("lollipop" or buccal tablet)	Actiq®, Fentora®
Hydromorphone (liquid, Injection, or suppository)	Dilaudid®
Meperidine (liquid or injection)	Demerol®
Oxycodone (liquid)	Oxydose®
Morphine (liquid, injections, or suppository)	Roxanol®
Oxymorphone (tablet)	Opana®
Hydrocodone (liquid)	Tussionex®

Rapid breakthrough pain relief within 5 to 15 minutes is the goal of the use of a breakthrough opioid medication. To achieve this rapid action, breakthrough opioids should be taken as a liquid, lollipop, injection, or suppository. They are commonly referred to as "short-acting" opioids because they may only act for one to three hours.

18. DON'T DEPEND ON ONE FAVORITE OPIOID OR ROUTE OF DELIVERY

One of the biggest mistakes an IP patient makes is to get too dependent on a favorite opioid such as fentanyl, meperidine, or oxycodone or the way it is delivered, such as an injection or lollipop. Why? You may eventually get tolerant to the opioid and must switch. Also, many are extremely expensive and health insurance plans simply will not pay for them. Their position is that the older generic opioids such as morphine, methadone, hydrocodone, meperidine, and hydromorphone are good enough for pain control.

You must identify several opioids that are effective for you. Do not plan on getting the one you most want. Cost factors have simply ushered in a situation that has priced some of the Step Two and break-through opioids out of range.

You should immediately look at the lists of opioids in this Handbook and determine which ones you have and have not tried. At a minimum, you should identify four that you can take, and which are effective. Also, do not get your heart set on route of administration such as a lollipop or injection. For survival, you must learn what your health plan will pay for. Do not expect your health plan to give you a special exception to their usual opioid and cost policy. It is usually a bad idea to take brand name opioids. Why? Sooner or later your health insurance will likely disallow brand names.

19. ANCILLARY MEDICATIONS

In addition to opioids, there are additional medications that almost all IP patients will require. One is a sleeping aid, and the other is a muscle relaxant. Hormone replacement of adrenal hormones, thyroid, estrogen, or testosterone may also be required as pain and/or opioid medications may deplete them. You may also need mediation for nausea, constipation, or weight control.

20. SLEEP

IP and its accompanying high pulse rate keep IP patients awake. You will likely need a sleep aid, and several of the favorites of IP patients are listed in the Table below. Some antidepressants, which activate serotonin are liked by patients and physicians because they assist sleep and depression at the same time. Furthermore, serotonin may promote neurogenesis or healing of nerves.

SOME SLEEP AIDS IP PATIENTS FIND EFFECTIVE	
AID	**COMMON TRADE NAME**
Chloral Hydrate	Somnote®
Triazolam	Halcion®
Temazepam	Restoril®
Zolpidem	Ambien®
Amitriptyline	Elavil®

IP patients all expect six to eight hours of sleep like a normal person. <u>DO NOT</u> expect this. You will likely not be able to sleep more than about four hours at a time. Many IP patients cannot sleep over two to three hours at a stretch. This is particularly true if you have damaged your spine, hips, knees, or nerves in your arms or legs. Why? If you sleep too long on these damaged tissues, you may crush them and produce more pain. Your body wants you to awake frequently so you avoid sleeping in one position and crush tissues which may increase your pain.

IP patients need to take their last daily opioid dose within one hour before bedtime. When you awake in the night, you should get out of bed, stretch, and use the restroom before returning to bed. If you have pain during the night, take a dose of your breakthrough opioid.

21. MUSCLE RELAXANT-ANTI-ANXIETY AGENTS

The severe pain and high pulse rate of IP causes anxiety and muscle contraction. A high pulse rate may make you feel jittery or nervous. In addition, you may have an injury that may cause muscle contraction. Most IP patients find that a muscle relaxant provides considerable additional pain relief and comfort. For reasons that are not particularly clear to me, some muscle relaxants are not effective in IP patients. Although pharmacologically classified as anti-anxiety agents, some are effective in reducing high pulse rates and muscle spasms. Those muscle relaxant-anti-anxiety agents that have proven to be popular with many IP patients are listed in the Table below. Do not take more than one of the agents in the Table on the same day. The #1 cause of sedation, falls, and accidents in IP patients is overdose of this group of agents.

MUSCLE RELAXANT ANTI-ANXIETY AGENTS	
AGENT	**COMMON TRADE NAME**
Carisoprodol	Soma®
Cyclobenzaprine	Flexeril®
Methocarbamol	Robaxin®
Diazepam	Valium®
Clonazepam	Klonopin®
Lorazepam	Ativan®

22. NERVE BLOCKERS

There are new drugs for pain relief that act by blocking the electricity in nerves. Pain that is caused by nerve damage in the legs, arm, chest wall, abdomen, or pelvis is often called "neuropathic pain." These agents can be used with opioids, and many patients can use these with a Step One opioid and avoid the necessity of Step Two opioids.

In milder forms of chronic pain, these agents may work so well that opioids are not even necessary. IP patients can sometimes reduce their opioid dosage with these agents. Some of the older anti-depressants and anti-seizure drugs are nerve blockers, and they have been extensively used for pain relief. The two newest on the market, however, are generally superior, and they are the only ones I now recommend.

NERVE BLOCKERS	
AGENT	**COMMON TRADE NAME**
Duloxetine	Cymbalta®
Pregabalin	Lyrica®

23. NUTRITIONAL AND HORMONAL AGENTS

IP patients must all take some nutritional and hormonal agents. IP depletes the body of certain nutritional substances and hormones. If these are depleted, pain worsens, and the patient will experience more fatigue, insomnia, and depression. IP patients should read about various dietary supplements and try ones that have an appeal. Currently, there is no marketed vitamin, mineral, herb, or amino acid that I restrict or condemn. Here are my minimal recommendations, for all IP patients.

1. Daily multiple-vitamin-mineral tablet or capsule.
2. Calcium, magnesium, and vitamin D. for osteoporosis prevention.
3. Pregnenolone 50 to 100mg a day. This is the basic adrenal hormone and nerve healer.

24. TOPICAL MEDICATIONS

To achieve better pain relief and promote healing, IP patients may find one or more topical medications which are rubbed into the skin over painful areas, to be effective. These agents are known as "topical" because they go on top of the skin. Since IP patients have tissue damage and scarring, internal medications may not always reach the damaged nerves because blood vessels in the damaged tissue area may also be damaged. Consequently, topical medications may be able to penetrate into damaged areas by diffusion.
The list of topical medications being used and researched throughout the country is too long to fully list here. IP patients are encouraged to ask their pharmacist or other IP patients if they recommend a specific topical medication. Then try it. Topical medications have essentially no permanent side effects, so you can experiment safely. The most consistent topical pain relievers in my experience have been morphine and carisoprodol. The formula is to crush tablets of medication and dissolve one or two tablets in one ounce of cold cream. Apply as often as necessary for pain control.

An excellent topical pain reliever is lidocaine, which is classified as a topical anesthetic. It is available as a patch (Lidoderm). This patch produces excellent pain relief for about twelve hours. It can be placed on the neck, back, hip, knee or other body area that is painful. Unless an IP patient has pain deep in the body such as abdominal adhesions, they can usually get good relief from the lidocaine patch. These patches are particularly effective if there is a pain flare or you have "overdone" it and caused some additional discomfort in a joint, back, or spine area by over-exercise.

25. CONSTIPATION

This troublesome problem often results from opioid drugs and inactivity. To help prevent it, drink six to eight glasses of fluids a day and take some fiber supplements which can be purchased over-the-counter at any grocery or drug store. Many over-the-counter laxatives are effective. I have not observed that one fiber product is superior to others. Therefore, it is a personal choice. I have surveyed patients repeatedly to determine a consensus on laxatives, but there is no agreement among IP patients as to which ones are best.

If fluids and non-prescription, over-the-counter laxatives do not do the job, there are several prescription laxatives. Simply ask a physician to give you a prescription. You may have to try several to settle on one you find most effective. I have found that my IP patients with severe constipation almost always respond to polyethylene glycol (GlycoLax®, MiraLax®, GoLYTELY®), or a licorice product called Evac-U- Gen®.

26. NEUROGENESIS: KEY TO CURE

Neurogenesis is the term used to mean new growth or regeneration of nerves. The key to cure or significant, permanent pain reduction of IP is neurogenesis – new nerve growth. A few years ago, it was believed that damaged nerves would not regrow. New research clearly shows that nerves can at least partially regrow. I have now witnessed so much permanent pain reduction in my IP patients that I believe permanent cure may even be possible for at least some patients, and permanent, partial pain reduction is possible in practically all IP patients.

Research on neurogenesis is starting to occur in a big way. IP patients should know that nerve growth is greatly dependent upon specific amino acids and hormones that promote nerve growth. Also, nerves probably can't regrow if pain is not well controlled because pain produces so much electrical activity in nerves that they cannot mend.

27. ANABOLIC THERAPY

Everyone is now familiar with "anabolic steroids" and the athletic advantage they provide by promoting muscle mass, speed, and endurance. The complications of over-bulking of tissue with anabolic steroids are also well known as too much bulk may injure knees, ankles, and joints. Anabolic steroids, when used in excess, can also produce cancer, heart disease, "roid rage," and impotence. These complications only occur, however, with mega-dosages that are clearly known to be dangerous.

What is important for every IP patient to know is that tissue regrowth and neurogenesis is enhanced by anabolic therapy. Anabolic simply means, from its Latin derivation," to promote growth." Therapeutic dosages of several anabolic, tissue-building agents are being studied in IP patients, and early research results are very promising. Listed here are some of the anabolic agents that I use in an attempt to promote growth of tissue, healing, and permanent pain reduction. This list is not complete and may not even contain the best agents, because many physicians are just now experimenting with many different anabolic approaches. I have only listed ones with which I am familiar and use. When prescribed by a knowledgeable physician, these agents are very safe and therapeutic. Other than some of the hormones, the other agents listed in the accompanying Table on Anabolic Agents can be purchased in health food stores, or through catalogues.

```
ANABOLIC AGENTS

HORMONES
Pregnenolone
Androstenedione
Testosterone
Dehydroepiandrosterone (DHEA
Chorionic Gonadotropin
Human Growth Hormone

AMINO ACIDS
Taurine
Glycine
Phenylalanine
Gamma Amino Butyric Acid

NERVE TISSUE BUILDER
Alpha Lipoic Acid
```

28. STRETCHING EXERCISES

Common strains and sprains that occur commonly with sports or excess physical activity tend to heal rapidly with repetitive motion and strengthening exercises. An example is lifting a weight several times to help heal and train an injured shoulder.

But IP patients are different and can even injure themselves if they participate or practice many of the exercises used for common strains and sprains. Why? IP results from nerve damage that is usually surrounded by scar tissue. Once IP and scarring has developed, one must be extremely cautious and careful when manipulating these tissue areas. For example, an exercise that suddenly pulls apart a scar may lead to additional scarring, nerve damage, and pain. Even if a damaged nerve wants to regrow, if it is trapped in a scar, new growth may not be possible. The reduction and elimination of scarring and the promotion of neurogenesis requires a special type of exercise known as "Stretch and Hold." These exercises are simple to execute.

Merely stretch your arm, leg, or spine to a point that you feel a tug or pull (not pain!!) at the painful site. Then hold the position for a count of fifteen to thirty seconds. Repeat this exercise a few times each day.

"Stretch and Hold" is designed to gently pull apart scars over time and lengthen the damaged areas so nerves can regrow.

DANGER: Do not do any exercise, physical therapy, gymnastics, or other activity that produces pain. Do not do any activity that increases your risk of tripping or falling.

REMEMBER: Pain is your enemy. If you cause it, you risk additional nerve damage to your already damaged area and you will age a little faster. As long as pain is not produced, you may do any physical activity you desire including swimming, bicycling, walking, sex, or treadmill.

29. DEALING WITH YOUR FAMILY AND LOVED ONES

IP is a family affair. In dealing with your family, your basic strategy is to discuss your situation honestly and openly. Do not be afraid to tell them about your true agony. Use information from this Handbook or other source. Your family first needs to know that IP is a rare condition and not the usual chronic pain of a bad back, arthritis, or TMJ. Educate yourself thoroughly about the Cardiac-Adrenal-Pain Syndrome and then pass on this information. Few people, including doctors, are yet aware of the seriousness of severe IP, and that if it is left uncontrolled, it will shorten life and produce serious complications.

Families who reject or do not believe IP is a serious disease and/or abhor the idea of opioid drugs must be dealt with firmly. They must be educated about the new research on cardiac and adrenal complications. If you have a family member(s) who rejects you or your treatment, you may need to notify them, in writing perhaps through your attorney, as to the nature of your condition and your necessity of opioid medications. More and more pain specialists are refusing to treat IP patients who do not have family support, because family members who dislike IP treatment frequently sue the patient's doctor after death or when a severe complication of IP such as dementia sets in. If you do not have a family member or spouse to advocate for you and be involved in your treatment program, you must find an advocate and confidant outside your immediate family who is going to be acquainted with your IP doctor and your situation. Do not be surprised if your IP doctor demands some legal protection or assurance from you that your family members will not sue him when you die or have a complication.

A problem sometimes encountered is that families do not understand an IP patient's need for rest and stress control. For example, too many people living and residing in the house of an IP patient may add to the stress of pain and further drive-up pulse rate and blood pressure. Your family needs to know what causes your pain to flare, so you can set up your daily living schedule and situation in such a manner as to minimize stress. Noise, crowding, offensive smells, or commotion may all stress an IP patient and worsen pain. You have to rid your house of obnoxious children and relatives.

30. WORK WITH YOUR HEALTH INSURANCE PLAN

Treatment of IP is intensive and expensive. Therefore, it behooves you to be extremely knowledgeable about your health plan. Here are the basics you must know:

1. What medications and number of monthly dosages will your plan cover? Obtain your Plan's formulary which lists the plan's drug benefits.

2. What doctors will your plan cover for your prescription drugs? Although you can likely afford to pay for a doctor visit out of your own pocket, the cost of IP treatment medications is so high that even very wealthy people cannot afford them. It is not uncommon for medication costs to run in the thousands of dollars each month.

3. Learn how to bill your plan for out-of-pocket costs. You and your family or non-family advocate must get on the phone or personally visit your plan's administrative offices to obtain its formulary, rules on doctor selection, and method for getting reimbursed for out-of-pocket costs. Some plans have their own reimbursement forms while others merely want a receipt. Many use the universal federal claim form.

4. Find out how to request medication that is not on your plan's formulary. In most cases, you will have to have tried all the formulary medications and dosages covered by your Plan before your Plan will allow exceptions. For starters, review the opioids listed in this Handbook. You will likely spot some you have never heard of but may be acceptable to you and your Plan.

The biggest problem with some Plans is that they try to force IP patients into detoxification or to reduce their medication. They often bad-mouth any doctor who adequately treats IP and tries to play up some doc who only prescribes aspirin or gives a nerve block. Make sure you know what happens to your pulse rate when you reduce your opioids. You could expire of a heart attack or stroke if you cut down too fast on your medication and your pain and pulse flare. You are particularly at risk if your pain has been well-controlled for several months. If you find yourself in a situation where your Plan may try to harm you by taking away your medication, you, and your advocate must personally – do not rely on your doctor or pharmacist – inform them about your condition and the cardiac risks of uncontrolled pain. Enlist your minister or other advocate. If your Plan does not listen, you will have to contact your State Insurance Complaint Agency. Almost all States now have these. Sadly, some IP patients have had to enlist the services of an attorney to force health plans to merely comply with their own stated and written benefits.

31. FINDING A DOCTOR TO TREAT IP

As of yet, few MD's in the United States specialize in IP. There is no Board certification for it, and no Family Practice or Internal Medicine Residency programs in universities offer fellowships in it. Most pain specialists in America are anesthesiologists. Most anesthesiologists, however, only perform interventions such as epidural nerve blocks or implant stimulators and do not medically manage IP over an extended period of time. IP patients throughout the country still have great difficulty obtaining enough opioids for proper pain control meaning the ability to regularly leave your home, have a quality of life, and keep pulse rate and blood pressure in normal range. Few family doctors or internists treat IP because the use of Step Two and breakthrough opioids are really the purview of the pain specialist.

IP patients frequently want their family doctor or internist to prescribe potent opioids, but the vast majority of primary care doctors should only prescribe Step One opioids. If you believe you have IP and require more opioids than you are able to obtain from your current MD's, you need to find a pain specialist who is qualified and knowledgeable about the Step Two and Breakthrough opioids. You may have to travel some distance, but IP patients need to be treated by a physician who not only can help you control IP but who wants to help you participate in neurogenesis and anabolic therapy, so you have an opportunity for possible cure or permanent reduction of pain.

To find a doctor, first try your health plan. Some are getting with the program and have MD's on their panels that treat IP. For the best sources, talk with IP patients who have been able to find the help they need.

32. STRESS CONTROL: MAINTAIN YOUR SPACE

Stress in an IP patient is anything that causes your pain to flare. This can be due to psychologic, financial, or marital conflicts. Anything that causes your heart to speed up will likely increase your pain. IP is the ultimate stress on the body, and even a little extra stress from another cause will increase pain and perhaps even add to the tissue damage that you have.

You must maintain your mental and physical space. You simply must get any nagging stress situation out of your life. This might be a marriage partner or a relative. For example, one of the greatest and most malignant stresses is a visitor to your home over a holiday or an unruly family member who lives with you. Whatever it takes, you must live and function in a peaceful, tranquil setting where you can come and go at your own pace. Stay out of situations such as jury duty or jobs which do not allow you to sit, stand, relax, or control your time.

33. TRAVEL AND WALKING TIPS

Many IP patients have been confined to home, bed, and couch, often for years. Now with opioid treatment they can travel and walk.

First bit of advice. Travel and walk every chance you get as long as it does not increase your pain. Plane, cruise, train, or bus. Go for it. Why? No one knows how long we will live, and this is particularly true of IP patients. It has only been in recent years that our governments – State and Federal – have allowed opioids to be used in the dosages that are truly effective and which will prolong an IP patient's life. But for how long? Without any treatment, IP patients die after only a few days or weeks following the start of IP. Now, however, IP patients may live almost a normal life span. I personally have IP patients who I have treated with high dose opioids for over twenty years. And they are still going strong with all their mental faculties. But do not count on a long future. Buy your travel ticket today!

Now for the do's and don'ts:

1. Do take your medication on a regular schedule even if you are on a plane, train, or ship.

2. Do not sit in a plane or car seat for more than thirty minutes at a stretch. Get up and stand or walk.

3. You cannot afford to fall or slip. Use a cane or walker if you are in unfamiliar territory.

4. If you have spine degeneration, you should wear a soft brace with shoulder straps when you fly or take a long car ride.

5. Carry a note from your doctor that states your problem and need for medication.

6. Hand-carry only the medication you need while flying. Pack the rest in a water-tight container in your suitcase. Critical: When traveling do not remove medication from the bottle or container that has a pharmacy label that shows your name, your doctor's name, and name of medication. If you remove your medication from its issued container and if authorities in an air or seaport find it, they will likely confiscate it as they should.

34. PREVENTING DEMENTIA AND MENTAL DETERIORATION

There is a dirty little secret about IP that no one wants to think about or talk about. Continuous, severe IP may cause brain atrophy. This fact has been scientifically proven by research with brain scans. It is believed to occur because pain is essentially an electric current. Consequently, it can literally burn tissue like any other over-electrified wire may burn out a socket or fuse. I call it the "hot-wire effect." Sort of like lightening striking you.

Every IP patient <u>MUST</u> embark on a mental protection plan. If you do not, you may sadly learn that your mental concentration, memory, and analytic skills may crumble. Reading, writing, and arithmetic may go downhill. But do not panic! Simply follow these guidelines.

1. Get maximal pain control. Pain is the enemy. Do not even let it flare if possible.

2. Hormone balance. Make sure your cortisol, pregnenolone, thyroid, and testosterone are normal.

3. Spend lots of time physically speaking and conversing with other people.

4. Read and write something every day. Watching TV will not get the job done. E-mail and chat rooms on the internet are terrific mental exercises.

5. Mental exercises. Crossword and jigsaw puzzles are thought by many clinicians to be excellent as dementia preventers. Any puzzles or games will do. Just keep your mind busy. Force yourself to do some arithmetic almost daily. Use it or lose it!

35. TOOTH DECAY AND OSTEOPOROSIS

IP, per se, causes several serious side effects. They primarily occur because IP may alter hormones produced by the pituitary and adrenal glands.

High cortisol (body's natural cortisone) causes a loss of calcium in bones and teeth. Consequently, your primary pain may be, for example, muscular, but your spine and teeth may degenerate. Or you may have an abdominal or spine condition and find that your knees deteriorate. In addition to hormone changes caused by pain, your teeth may deteriorate due to pain causing you to hold your mouth in an abnormal position and cause your breathing to be altered. Saliva production is also altered in IP. IP causes insulin to rise and blood sugar to lower, which in turn causes IP patients to crave sugars and starches, which may harm teeth. Your mouth contains good and bad bacteria, and IP causes changes in your immune system. Lastly, some pain medications may contain sugar which accelerates tooth decay, and they may interfere with bone and teeth growth.

All in all, almost every IP patient will suffer tooth decay and require fillings and tooth extractions. Osteoporosis can be so serious in IP patients that spines and joints can severely degenerate and collapse.

Consequently, IP patients must develop a program to prevent tooth decay and osteoporosis. Here are measures you must take to best reduce the severity of tooth decay and osteoporosis:

1. Keep your pain controlled so that your pulse, blood pressure, and hormone, blood levels are normal.

2. Brush and/or floss teeth daily and rinse often with a mouth wash. Vigorous, periodic, dental cleaning by your dentist may help.

3. Reduce sugars in your diet, particularly drinks that contain carbohydrates (sugars). Follow the nutritional guidelines in this Handbook .

4. Take these supplements daily:

   Calcium – 1000 to 1200mg
   Vitamin D – 600 units
   Magnesium – 500mg

36. POTENTIATORS: WHAT ARE THEY?

The term "potentiator" is one used by physicians and pharmacists to indicate that one medical agent makes another more "potent." Here, we are talking about agents that make opioids act stronger and last longer. Potentiators allow less opioid to be used and lessen their complications. In this day and age of cost cutting most IP patients will have to learn to use potentiators because insurance plans will not pay for the most effective opioids.

Additionally, when you wish to decrease your opioids or attempt to withdraw, you will need to use a lot of potentiators. Common agents which potentiate opioids, and which are commercially placed in some opioids are: Caffeine, Aspirin, Acetaminophen, and Ibuprofen. For example, Vicodin®, Percocet®, and Darvocet® contain acetaminophen. Fiorinal® contains caffeine and aspirin. Vicoprofen® contains ibuprofen.

Other agents including some muscle relaxants and stimulants potentiate opioids. IP patients should take a variety of potentiators to determine which ones make your opioid more effective. IP patients must especially learn to take a potentiator with their breakthrough opioids since a potentiator can help break a flare. Here is a partial list of some potentiators which may boost your breakthrough opioid: Caffeine Tablet, Dexedrine, Acetaminophen, Phentermine, Midrin®, Aspirin.

You should systematically try potentiators one at a time to determine how best to control breakthrough pain without the benefit of expensive commercial opioid preparations such as fentanyl (Actiq® or Fentora®).

37. THE TYLENOL® PROBLEM

Tylenol® is acetaminophen. It is an effective opioid potentiator, and it is found in many popular opioid formulations (see Table).

OPIOID	COMMON TRADE NAMES
Hydrocodone	Vicodin®, Lortab®, Norco®
Oxycodone	Percocet®
Tramadol	Ultracet®
Propoxyphene	Darvocet®
Codeine	Empirin®

As long as patients do not take over about 4000mg a day of acetaminophen, it is safe to take. Acetaminophen daily dosages above 4000mg a day may cause liver or kidney toxicity. The maximal dose of Norco®, for example, is twelve tablets a day.

IP patients should know which opioid-acetaminophen combination works for them. The combination agents are relatively safe and inexpensive as long as the 4000mg a day level is not exceeded. When an IP patient wishes to reduce or withdraw from Step Two opioids, they should switch from a pure opioid drug such as hydromorphone (Dilaudid®), Oxycodone (OxyContin®), or methadone (Dolophine®) to a Step One opioid that contains acetaminophen.

38. DIET: PROTEIN IS YOUR BEST FRIEND

Protein is comprised of about twenty-five different amino acids. The body takes amino acids and uses them individually or in a grouping (i.e., molecule) for various pain control functions.

For example, endorphin, which is the body's natural pain reliever, is a grouping of about seventeen of the twenty-five amino acids. There are at least six single amino acids that the body uses for specific functions to control pain. Shown here is a Table of these because IP patients must eat some protein foods to obtain enough amino acids for the body to effectively control pain. Do not expect your prescription opioids and other medications to work very well if you do not take in enough protein or amino acid supplements. Amino acids can be purchased in most any health food store or through catalogs.

SINGLE AMINO ACID	PAIN CONTROL FUNCITON
Gamma Amino Butyric Acid	Prevents pain transmission along nerves.
Glycine	Activates pain control in the spinal cord.

Taurine	Activates pain control centers (receptors) in brain and spinal cord.
Phenylalanine & Tyrosine	Produces adrenalin, noradrenalin, and dopamine that control stress, and provides energy, fights fatigue, and prevents depression.
Tryptophan	Produces serotonin which promotes sleep, enhances self-esteem, and prevents depression.

Please note the above list does not include vegetables or nuts. Why? While some vegetables and nuts contain as much as 30% protein, they will not, by themselves, suffice to meet the amino acid requirements of an IP patient.

Early morning is the most important time of day to eat protein. If you prime your body with protein early in the day, you give your body enough amino acids to allow your opioids and other medications to optimally work. Early morning protein is also a key to weight control. Simply put, you must prime your body each morning with protein. You should consume protein within two hours after you awake each morning.

PROTEIN FOODS

An IP patient needs to eat some protein 3 times aday. Here is a list of protein foods which is de- fined as over 50% protein by weight:

Chicken	Turkey	Beef
Cheese	Pork	Fish / Seafood
Lamb	Eggs	Cottage Cheese

What if you just cannot stand protein foods or eating early in the morning? Get over it. Think of early morning protein as a medicine, not food. Forget the taste – go for the medicinal value. As a substitute or partial substitute for protein foods, you can obtain the amino acids you require by using protein powders, capsules, or drinks which you can purchase from about any pharmacy or health food store. Just make sure you take them early each morning.

Another thing to consider is cholesterol and triglycerides. Sugars, starches, and fats are all converted by the body to cholesterol and triglycerides. While the fat in beef or bacon will raise triglycerides there is little fat in chicken or fish. The cholesterol in eggs is dissolved by stomach acid, so the scare over eggs causing your cholesterol to rise is a myth. Poor pain control raises your cholesterol and triglycerides because severe pain causes the adrenal glands to secrete excess cortisol. Although research is early, the high levels of cholesterol and triglycerides found in IP patients undoubtedly causes heart and stroke complications.

39. WEIGHT GAIN

Unless you take extraordinary measures, you will gain excess weight after you develop IP. Not only do you face all the great foods and life-style attractions that fatten up about everyone in modern day society, IP has some other complications that cause obesity.

1. IP causes a change in insulin and blood sugar levels that make you only want to eat sugars and starches (carbohydrates) at the expense of protein.

2. Most causes of IP slow movement and restrict exercise, so you cannot burn fat very well.

3. Almost all medications used for pain treatment slow metabolism and produce weight gain. These include opioids, anti-depressants, sleep aids, muscle relaxants, anti-anxiety drugs, and nerve block agents.

There is no guarantee that weight reduction will reduce your pain, particularly if your pain is caused by headaches, adhesions, fibromyalgia, or nerve damage in your arms, legs, chest wall, or pelvis. But if your pain is caused by spine or joint degeneration, you will likely have less pain and need less medication for pain control if you lose just a few pounds.

Your first and most critical step in weight reduction is to <u>stop all table sugar and liquids that contain carbohydrates</u>. This includes milk, regular sodas, fruit juices and the so-called "energy drinks." Look at the label of everything you drink. The label should say: "carbohydrates - 0." Table sugars and liquids cause your blood sugar to rise so fast that about two hours later you get a rebound low blood sugar, (hypoglycemia) that makes you crave even more sugars and starches. One major key to weight reduction is to reduce sugars and starches and replace them with protein foods

Some IP patients who lose only three to five pounds reduce their pain. This is particularly true if your pain is due to <u>spine, hip, or knee degeneration</u>.

A mild stimulant is a big help. Caffeine is one of the best. In the case of an IP patient, you can hardly overdo caffeine. Drink all the tea, coffee, and diet drinks with caffeine you can stand! Caffeine not only helps weight reduction, but it is an opioid potentiator. Some IP patients benefit from an appetite suppressant such as phendimetrazine, phentermine, or Dexedrine. Not only will these agents help control weight, but they also act as opioid potentiators and decrease any sedation your medication may cause.

40. KNOW YOUR CAUSE AND ATTACK IT

When you develop IP, you do not much care about its underlying cause, or what is causing anyone else's pain. This is a mistake. You should learn all about the basic cause(s) of your pain. Read about it. Join the advocacy group or groups that champion and advocate for research on your specific cause of pain. Some excellent examples are fibromyalgia, reflex sympathetic dystrophy, interstitial cystitis, abdominal adhesions, and vulvodynia. Keep up on the latest scientific advances. If you hear or think of anything that might help your underlying cause, bring it to your doctor's attention. Always keep trying to cure or ameliorate your underlying cause. In addition to your pain doctor, you should have a doctor who specializes in your underlying disease.

41. PAIN RELIEF FOR SURGERY OR DENTAL PROCEDURES

In the event you must have surgery or dental procedures, there are certain do's and don'ts. Please let your surgeon or dentist know about the recommendations listed here.

1. Take your regular medications, particularly your long-acting opioid, on your regular daily schedule up to and immediately after the procedure. DO NOT alter your regular, usual daily medication regimen, before the surgery.

2. For extra pain relief during and after the procedure you will need to DO one of two things:

   a. Take an increased amount of your short-acting or breakthrough opioid.

b. Your surgeon or dentist can give you a very-short acting opioid by injection or suppository if the procedure causes a severe pain flare. EXAMPLES: meperidine (Demerol®) injection, or hydromorphone (Dilaudid®) injection or suppository. In addition, you may find that an oral, Step One opioid such as Vicodin® or Panlor® is very helpful.

42. CUTTING DOWN AND WITHDRAWING FROM OPIOIDS

Once an IP patient has taken opioids long enough to have some pain free hours each day, it is time to attempt dosage reduction. <u>Do not try to reduce opioid dosage until you have some pain free hours.</u> When you achieve some pain free hours, it means that some neurogenesis or healing has been achieved, and you probably do not need as much medication.

When you start reducing medication, I recommend you reduce 5% to 10% a week. For example, if you take ten morphine pills a day reduce your dose to nine for one week. Then a week later you can go down another pill each day. Try to withdraw over a three to four-month period. If you withdraw too fast, you may cause a severe pain flare which may set you back or make you worse.

Every IP patient will encounter someone in their life - be it a spouse, pharmacist, minister, doctor, friend, or relative - who will try to talk you into stopping your medication. Do not be foolish. Review the complications of IP. If you must, simply take your opioids for the remainder of your life. Just do not fall for some ignorant or fraudulent line that you should stop your medication, as long as you have pain.

If you still have pain and decide to go into a detox center to stop your drugs, do not expect your pain doctor to either approve or take you back as a patient. Why? Either you have IP and need medication, or you do not. Remember, detox centers are for addicts, not legitimate pain patients. If you let anyone – spouse, psychiatrist, minister, or pharmacist – talk you into stopping medication, just remember that there are several tombstones in the cemetery that are there because an IP patient stopped their drugs too abruptly and caused a severe pain flare and heart stoppage.

Here are absolute DON'TS:

1. Do not try to withdraw from medication until you have at least some pain free hours each day. Until you have pain-free hours you have too much nerve damage to reduce pain control medications.

2. Do not believe any claim that your medication is causing your pain or that pain will be gone if you suddenly stop your medication.

3. Do not withdraw rapidly. Lower your dose 5% to 10% a week, and simply return to your regular daily dose or hold your dosage at a lowered level if your pain resumes.

4. Do not let anybody put you in a hospital to "detoxify" or take you off your medication. Do it slowly over three to four months in your own home environment. Withdraw at a speed that does not cause your pain to flare.

There is a good way to get off opioids or to lower your dose. Once you have lowered your daily dose, switch to a milder, Step One opioid which has acetaminophen in it. Try one of the new nerve blockers such as duloxetine (Cymbalta®), and a muscle relaxant. Stay on this regimen for two to three months and then reduce these medications. Your doctor can probably assist with some other withdrawal tips and medications. Biggest tip: many chronic disease patients such as diabetics must take medication all their life; if this is necessary, simply continue taking your pain medication – you do not have to stop.

43. INTERVENTIONS – A NEW TERM IN PAIN TREATMENT

The term "intervention" is used to describe a set of procedures that may permanently or temporarily reduce the severity of your pain. Some anesthesiologists and rehab physicians now refer to themselves as "Interventional Pain Specialists." These physicians primarily specialize in medical procedures involving the spine. Consequently, if you have spine degeneration as the cause of your pain, you should see an interventional pain specialist to determine if there is a procedure that can help you.

Once you get your pain under control with opioids and other measures listed in this Handbook, you should consider the procedures and interventions that modern medicine has to offer. For example, injections in or around the spine, laser, Botox®, or prolotherapy may permanently reduce some of your pain. The very best time to try interventions, including surgery, is when your pain is under control. Why?

Controlled pain means your hormones and immune system are in good shape to help you heal. Many IP patients often believe that procedures or interventions they attempted in the past won't work in the future. This may not be true since efforts in the past were likely attempted when pain was not controlled. Sometimes it pays handsomely to try again.

There are two cardinal rules. Do not attempt an intervention that causes pain. Simply stop in the middle of the procedure if necessary.

The second is don't stop your medication to try a procedure or intervention. Only an ignorant or biased practitioner will even suggest you stop your medication to have surgery or an intervention. Turn and run from any practitioner who may suggest this.

44. OPIOID PUMPS AND ELECTRICAL STIMULATORS

Interventional pain doctors now specialize in implanting opioid pumps and electrical stimulators in the spinal cord. Opioid administration directly into the spinal cord is called "intrathecal administration." If you find you cannot adequately control your pain with the Step One, Step Two, and Breakthrough Opioids listed in this Handbook, you should consider an implanted intrathecal device. These implanted devices by-pass the stomach and liver to place opioids directly into brain fluids. Often times pain relief, by this procedure, is far superior to other methods of administration. In addition, there is a new medication called ziconotide (Prialt®), which is not an opioid, but provides great pain control and can only be taken through an implanted intrathecal device.

Another successful implant is known as a "spinal cord stimulator." These devices send a special kind of electrical signal into the spinal cord and nerves that go into the legs and arms. Particularly with some cases of reflex sympathetic dystrophy and neuropathies, these new stimulators may provide excellent relief.

While no one likes the idea of an implanted device, the modern implants can often provide excellent pain relief. Be honest with yourself. If medical management is not getting the job done for you, ask one of your physicians to refer you to an "Interventional Pain Specialist." In most cases these interventionalist pain doctors can test you ahead of time to see if the implant will work so you do not have to risk a procedure. IP patients who have implants still have to take other medications including opioids. Do not fall for any line that an implant will totally substitute for your current opioid medication. You may be able to reduce your medications with an implant, but implants will not totally substitute your need for medication. Be advised that these implants are quite expensive, and your health plan may resist paying for them.

45. HORMONE REPLACEMENT AND TREATMENTS

Hormone treatment along with good pain control, protein diet, stretching exercises, and positive mental attitude give you the best hope for neurogenesis and permanent healing. Replacement means that you take hormones that are depleted by pain and/or medications. Be clearly advised that a most serious complication of opioids is hormone depletion, particularly testosterone. You will need a blood test to determine whether this is the case. Testosterone, in males and females, is necessary for good pain control, energy, weight control, bone growth, libido, and relief of depression.

Severe IP may deplete certain pituitary and adrenal hormones. Although research on hormones is in its early stage, I have found that the adrenal hormone, pregnenolone, is almost always depleted by IP. This hormone naturally acts to heal nerves and promote energy and mental ability. Patients who don't have enough pregnenolone are depressed, exhausted, have poor mental concentration, memory, and pain control. If you have IP, I recommend a daily dose of 50 to 200mg. The only known side effect of these dosages is acne, and if this occurs, reduce your dosage. Some IP patients appear to have inadequate thyroid or estrogen levels. You may need to be tested for these hormones and take replacements. Some hormones such as chorionic gonadotropin and growth hormone cause tissue growth (i.e., "anabolic effect") and appear to offer hope in permanently reducing IP.

46. QUALITY OF LIFE

Make a better quality of life your number two priority after you get some pain relief. You will find it a tough job. Chances are you will always have the pain nagging at you, and you may have spent so much time in bed or on the couch that you have forgotten how to socialize and communicate with the outside world. You may also have spent so much time wallowing in your self-pity that you have forgotten how to be a friend to anyone. Pain robs one of interest in much else besides relief. With opioids and reduced pain, you MUST start communicating and talking with other people. You simply have to go visit, call on the phone, and talk with live people. In this situation, e-mails and chat rooms on the internet will not entirely cut it. Talk is therapy for a pain patient.

You will need some at-home hobbies or activities. Something that you enjoy and that at least partially takes your mind off your pain. Work for pay or volunteer. Drive a car if at all possible.

You will need to come to grips with your religious beliefs. Most patients with IP have either thought about suicide or come close to death. Some have had near death experiences or technically died and come back. Regardless of your particular situation, please give prayer and your church your best effort with time and thought. Remember. Your survival instinct, attitude, and modern medicine have given you a lease on life, and your God still wants you here on earth for some purpose that only you know.

47. PLANTS, PETS, AND MUSIC

You need all three. There is something about live DNA
around you that is a great comfort. Make no mistake. Pets like a dog
or cat who is attached to you will literally know when you are in pain.
Sometimes they will know you are about to have a flare before you
do!

Plants cannot speak or cuddle up to you, but I know this. IP patients
who keep a lot of those green, leafy, colored jewels in pots around
the house or lawn just do a lot better with pain control. Your favorite
music is known to activate endorphins. No wonder some pain
patients find considerable comfort when they listen to their favorite
songs. Play it again, SAM! Better yet, drag out the old piano or violin
if you used to play.

48. GETTING YOUR MEDICATIONS IN THE HOSPITAL

If you are hospitalized either for an emergency or for a planned
surgery, you must be prepared for the hospital to deprive you of your
usual medications. Remember: Few hospital personnel are aware or
have even seen a bona fide IP case who legitimately requires a high
daily opioid dosage. Chances are that some well-meaning nurse will
confiscate your regular medication, and you may not get it back. At
all times, including a stay in the hospital, protect your supply of
medications. To ensure that you get your regular pain relief regimen
in the hospital, discuss your concerns and fears with your doctor
before you enter the hospital. Never try to hide your problem or be
ashamed of any medication you must take.

If you find yourself in a hospital and cannot obtain your usual pain
medications, your family and advocates will have to call on the

hospital administrator. You will probably find that the hospital administrator will be much more attuned to your problem than most of the nurses. Inform the administrator of your risks for a heart attack or stroke if your pain flares. Make it clear that you have legal rights to receive your usual medications while in the hospital.

49. YOU NEED A MINISTER AND LAWYER

Every IP patient should inform their minister of their situation. Many times, your clergyman can help you obtain services or assistance you may need. Above all, I recommend you strive to develop a good understanding of your illness and how it relates to your chosen religion.

You need a lawyer who is familiar with the laws and rights of IP patients. If you have a family attorney, give him or her the laws and materials about IP that you have accumulated. Many IP patients have had to use an attorney to obtain the help they need, such as obtaining disability benefits or forcing your health plan to provide the services they have promised.

One strategy I recommend is to join Pre-Paid Legal. This organization is a type of HMO for legal problems. You pay a small fee each month. When you have a legal problem, you will have excellent service that is already pre-paid. Since, IP patients all over the country are being bombarded with legal issues, you need to be ready if you develop a legal problem obtaining physician services or medications.

50. ADVOCACY GROUPS

Every IP patient should join one or more pain advocacy groups. Plenty are listed on the internet. Dues are nominal. And after you join, educate the group about your own case including difficulties in obtaining care, haggles with health plan coverage, and the serious cardiac and adrenal complications of IP. I know of no organization that specializes in finding physicians for IP patients.

51. HUMOR AND MOTIVATION – KEEP SMILING

To survive you need to keep a sense of humor and motivation. A smile, chuckle, or laugh actually stimulates the body's natural pain and immune systems to positively react. Whatever you can do to "keep smiling" must be done whether it is reading the funnies, visiting friends, or playing with your pet.

You must stay motivated to improve your situation. Do not necessarily be motivated to "beat it." If you are even reading this Handbook, chances are you have too much nerve damage to "beat it." Stay motivated to constantly improve your quality of life, minimize your pain, and promote neurogenesis.

52. SELF CHECK FOR OVER-MEDICATION

When your dosage of medications is proper, regardless of how high your dosage may be, you should not be sedated or impaired. Check out these indicators at home.

1. Can you walk upstairs without tripping?

2. Can you walk around your yard and neighborhood?
3. Can you read a newspaper or magazine?
4. Can you do simple mathematics?

You should train persons who live with you, particularly your primary advocate, to observe you for slurred speech, droopy eyes, sleepy appearance, and slow walking. They need to let you know if they believe you are over-medicated. You may not want to hear this message, but you must take corrective measures. If you take too much medication your pulse rate and blood pressure will be:

- Pulse below 72 per minute.
- Blood pressure below 120/80 mm/Hg.

If your dosage is proper and pain is controlled, you can drive a car and do paid or volunteer work. Do anything you wish as long as it does not cause your pain to flare.

53. KEEP A ONE WEEK RESERVE OF MEDICATION

It is critical that every IP patient keep at least a one-week reserve supply of all medication at all times. You are foolish to ever use up your total supply. Why? Doctors and pharmacies are highly regulated by the government and most doctors have to submit special, written prescriptions to obtain the controlled drugs necessary for IP control. This may require a few days. What if your doctor is not available? Only a few doctors will prescribe opioid drugs since they are risky and dangerous. What if there's a natural disaster such as an earthquake, fire, or tornado? Today, insurance companies will usually only pay for a thirty-day supply. This means you will have to put aside a reserve out of your usual monthly allotment. No matter. Keep in mind that the most common reason to use up your reserve is a medical emergency such as a dental abscess, or accident which may cause you to have a severe pain flare.

54. NEVER RUN OUT OF MEDICATION

Never call your doctor and ask for an early refill of your medication. Why? You destroy your relationship with not only your doctor, but likely with your pharmacist and health plan. If your doctor is in a group, one call for an early refill may get you labeled as a "trouble-making drug abuser." If you cannot manage your medication between doctor visits, you will likely soon find yourself without a pain doctor. If you need more medication or a higher dosage to help you control your pain between doctor visits, explain this to your spouse or the family member or supporter who you confide in and rely on. Then you and your advocate should jointly inform your doctor of your needs. Make sure this is a seldom event.

Know this... IP patients who ask for early refills or constantly change medication or dosage will be looked at by their doctor, pharmacist, or insurance plan as a drug abuser or, worse, someone who sells part of their drug supply. Doctors can rarely refill your medication before time or change dosages or brands between clinic visits. If you know your doctor very well and he knows you, he can do this on occasion. But do not expect it with controlled drugs.

55. YOUR MEDICAL RECORDS AND MRI'S

To get enough medications and help to survive, you T have in your possession your key, past medical records, and any MRI's you may have had on your spine, knees, hips, or other damaged areas. Same for your past laboratory results and physician evaluations. Never depend upon some image center, hospital, lab, or doctor to maintain your records and MRI's. Why? Do not expect any insurance company to pay for medication, much less be granted disability benefits, unless you can produce your past records and MRI's. A picture says a thousand words. Requests from IP patients for disability, medical procedures, and medication are routinely rejected, dismissed, and denied because no insurance company or government agency willingly spends money unless you have photographic proof of injury and medical records that document your case.

The most critical reason to keep medical records is to document that your pain is legitimate, incurable, and that you have had multiple physicians evaluate and treat you. Most State IP laws require that IP be documented and that can only be done with medical records from multiple sources.

56. DON'T BE A SOAP OPERA

What is a soap opera known for? One crisis after another, usually caused by the ignorance and apathy of the show's pathetic characters. Some IP patients have one crisis after another due to their basic personality or they have learned to create one crisis after another to gain attention, sympathy, or treatment. However, do not pull this act on a good pain doctor very often, because sooner or later he will discharge you. Why? Only patients who demonstrate responsibility and stability can legally and ethically be trusted with the potentially dangerous and abusable controlled drugs which are required to treat IP. Physicians are ethically and legally required to prevent diversion and abuse of controlled drugs. If you cannot control your life and live from crisis to crisis your doctor should say bye-bye. You would be shocked to hear all the reasons a pain doctor hears from patients for missed appointments, failure to obtain laboratory tests, dosage changes, and consultations. My cat is sick, car will not run, third cousin died, mail was late, lost my appointment card, house was robbed, toilet backed up, stuck a toothpick in my foot, etc., etc.

As an IP patient you must live in a stable, quiet environment. Here are some <u>MUSTS</u>.

1. Arrange your finances and insurance to obtain treatment.
2. Find one pharmacy and laboratory for your medications and tests.
3. Your living quarters must be free of commotion, loud noise, and too many inhabitants. Kick all drug abusers out of your house.
4. Your living quarters must be clean and orderly.
5. Arrange for regular meals and transportation.
6. Settle family and marital discord by whatever means it takes including separation and divorce.
7. Arrange to safely store your medications away from children, animals, and visitors.
8. You must develop activities, hobbies, crafts, or other endeavors to occupy your time.
9. Dress and act responsibly and kindly in public. If you look and act like a street or homeless person, your doctor might not keep you as a patient.
10. Do not use any illegal substances such as marijuana or drugs bought off the internet or from a foreign country.

Be clearly advised that your pain doctor will consider you irresponsible and list you on his potential discharge list if you do any of the following:

- Lose your medication.
- Constantly want your dosage or medication changed.
- Repeatedly miss appointments.
- Fail to obtain tests or follow orders and advice.
- Refuse to take urine, blood, or other tests.
- Look irresponsible.

Also be advised; pain doctors are taught in their seminars to reject patients if they do any of the above. Most pain doctors keep a mental or actual written list of problem patients who may require discharge. So many family members of IP patients have brought malpractice suits against pain doctors, and so many drug abusers manipulate doctors that you and your family must demonstrate stability and responsibility to stay off the "potential discharge list."

An IP patient needs to develop an attitude and life program to not only eliminate crises, but a planned program of progressive happiness and joy. Just because you have pain does not preempt you from improving your self-esteem, joy, and love for others. Even more important is that a positive mental attitude and constantly improving quality of life helps build your internal neurotransmitters and immune systems that promote neurogenesis and permanent pain reduction.

57. APPLYING FOR DISABILITY OR WORKER'S COMPENSATION

IP patients tend to have a terrible failing. They believe instinctively that they are so miserable and hurt so bad that they should automatically be awarded disability or worker's compensation benefits. Further-more, they tend to believe that other people recognize their plight and will be sympathetic. Another serious misconception is that they believe physician pain specialists can easily secure IP patient's disability or worker's compensation benefits because only a worthy, needy, truly deserving person would be under the care of a pain specialist. Wrong!

Here are the facts. Government and other agencies who award benefits do not believe anybody and have little sympathy simply because they are constantly lied to. Your pain doctor may have little say, because all kinds of charlatans who call themselves "doctors" constantly bombard the disability and worker's compensation systems with false or misleading information. Included in this group are a lot (not all) chiropractors, physical therapists, psychologists, and rehab counselors.

The first thing you must do to obtain disability or worker's compensation benefits is to obtain a comprehensive set of your medical records. You will primarily need records from doctors and hospitals who initially diagnosed and treated your injury or disease that caused your pain. Records from your pain doctor showing you have pain and need treatment are secondary.

If you plan to apply for disability, sit right down and make a list of the doctors, clinics, and hospitals you saw when you first developed your pain. Even though records of your initial problem may be several years old, they help make your case. After you make your list and obtain the records, your IP doctor can assist with the proper application. All you need is the name and address of the doctors, clinics, and hospitals you have seen.

Do not ask your IP doctor or his staff to get names, addresses, and zip codes of your previous medical care. This is your job. Once you put together a good set of medical records, your pain doctor and other current MD's you see can help prepare reports or complete forms for you.

You will need one other thing: a lawyer who specializes in obtaining benefits. To find one, ask other IP patients for a referral. Most attorneys who do this type of work wait until you are awarded benefits before you pay attorney fees. Do not try to apply for disability or worker's compensation benefits without an attorney. The disability and worker's compensation systems are so complex and assaulted by so many fraudulent persons and practitioners that you will need a competent, knowledgeable, professional to tackle the system.

58. SELECTING AND TRAINING YOUR PHARMACIST

The cardinal rule in dealing with pharmacies and pharmacists is to know that many, if not most, do not stock the drugs required to treat IP. Remember, true IP is a rare condition. Your pharmacy must be able to do the following:

1. Stock your medication.
2. Willing to communicate with your pain doctor.
3. Mail medications to you in an emergency.
4. Bill your insurance plan.
5. Apply for any exceptions to your health plan's formulary.

Pharmacies throughout the country are now willing and able to serve IP patients. Simply ask your pain doctor or other IP patients whom they recommend. Some specialize in pain treatment.

The first thing you need to do is take the pharmacy a note from your pain doctor telling the pharmacy the cause of your pain and what general treatment (i.e., opioids, ancillary medications, etc.) you will require. Ideally, this note should be on your doctor's stationary in order to give the pharmacy your doctor's address, phone, and fax.

Second, to help, give your pharmacy the following list of terms and abbreviations: IP = Intractable Pain; CP = Chronic Pain; BTP = Breakthrough Pain; EPR = Emergency Pain Relief; MS = Muscle Spasm; AP = Acute Pain

Lastly, keep your pharmacist informed. Drop off any literature or written materials you come across regarding IP. Pharmacists have a grapevine better than Ma Bell, and they are doing great service to all parties by their education efforts regarding pain.

59. THE DRUG VICES: ALCOHOL, MARIJUANA, NICOTINE, COCAINE, AND METHAMPHETAMINE

If you have IP and need long-term opioid therapy, heed carefully this section.

Almost all overdoses and deaths in IP patients happen, not because of legitimate medications, but the patient drank too many alcoholic beverages or used other, non-prescribed chemicals. Also, be clearly advised, that ethical pain physicians cannot condone the use of any illegal substance including marijuana, cocaine, methamphetamine, and drugs purchased off the internet or from foreign countries. Most pain doctors now periodically test their patients for illegal drugs by urine or blood. If you are asked to test and fail to cooperate, expect your pain doctor to give you the old heave ho. And if you test positive for any illegal substance, do not expect your pain doctor to keep you. Why? Legal and ethical liability. In addition, use of the vice-drugs may interfere with pain medication meaning that their effectiveness is diminished.

Limit alcohol to two small drinks a day. Even this amount may be too much if your advocates and family say it impairs you. Be advised that alcohol taken with acetaminophen compounds accelerate liver damage. Excess alcohol taken with aspirin and anti-inflammatory agents causes stomach bleeding and ulcers.

Nicotine does not directly interfere with pain treatment. Heavy smoking may be hazardous in IP patients above its well-known cancer, emphysema, and heart affects, by lowering your immune and healing capability. Patients who have a painful condition that diminishes their breathing capacity should limit smoking. All anti-smoking patches and medications can be taken with pain treatment medication.

57

60. OVERDOSE DEATHS: WHY DOCTORS ARE STOPPING PAIN PRACTICE

Be clearly advised that physicians all over the country are dropping the care of pain patients due to the misuse of drugs by pain patients. I have reviewed numerous malpractice cases where the doctor is charged with substandard practice.

Overdose deaths are the major problem, and the overdose is almost always due to a patient who consumed drugs other than as prescribed. The number one cause of overdose death is the patient who takes too many muscle relaxants such as Soma® with another anti-anxiety drug, such as Valium® or Ativan®. Rather than take the risks, many doctors are just saying no to pain patients. You can help. Do not take drugs other than as prescribed. Do not give away or sell your drugs. Most of all do not take more than one muscle relaxant and sedative on the same day.

61. MILESTONE: PAIN FREE HOURS

The hallmark of IP is constancy of the pain. It is always present when you are awake. It is caused by nerve damage somewhere in the body. Once you are in treatment and achieving good pain control, your damaged nerves should undergo at least some neurogenesis (nerve growth). You will know this is happening when you find that you have some hours in which you simply do not have pain, or very little. When you finally achieve the milestone of some pain free hours each day or week, you will know you are not just surviving but starting to thrive. Stay the course. You have achieved a major milestone, and many more will come.

62. APPENDIX

Appendix A. Inventory of Pain Triggers

Ask yourself which of the following triggers makes your pain start or flare?

Sitting in one place for more than ten minutes
Standing in one spot for over three minutes
Getting in or out of bed
Getting in or out of a car
A long car or plane ride
Doing household chores more than fifteen minutes
Working on your car for over five minutes
Doing yardwork for over five minutes
Walking for ten minutes
Shopping for thirty minutes
Writing for five minutes
Reading over ten minutes
Skipping breakfast
Skipping lunch or dinner
A poor night's sleep
Rainy or foggy weather
Hot weather
Cold weather
Conversation with certain people
Shower or bath
Loud noise
Visits with certain relatives or friends
Sexual relations
Argument with family members
Argument with non-family persons
Eating certain foods (which ones?)
Drinking caffeine
Drinking alcohol

Applying cosmetics, lotion, or medicine to skin
Listening to unpleasant music
Being in a situation where you can't sit or lie down
Driving a car
Working too many hours
Wearing certain clothes or shoes
Standing or stretching in certain position
Getting angry or mad at someone
Parties/holiday festivities
Family reunion

Appendix B. Inventory of Pain Relievers

Ask yourself which of the following relieves some of your pain?

Hot water bottle or heating pad
Ice packs
Bengay® or other topical ointment
Back brace
Knee brace
Cane
Support shoes
Arch supports
Aspirin
Acetaminophen (Tylenol®)
Caffeine (coffee, tea, soda drinks)
Ibuprofen
Naprosyn®
Naps or rests during the day
Eating breakfast
Walking
Stretching arms
Stretching legs
Stretching back

Stretching neck
Petting/cuddling an animal
Massaging painful area
Continuous sleep for four or more hours
Watching a movie
Attend church
Praying
Visit with friend
Visit with family
Visit with children
Reading for fifteen or more minutes
Watching television
Gardening or plant care
Relieve constipation
Drink alcohol
Swim or walk in water
Hot bath or shower
Vitamin/mineral tablets
Amino acids
Herbs
Crossword puzzle
Jigsaw puzzle
Losing five pounds of weight
Drive a car
Listen to your favorite music

Appendix C. Nutrition Measures to Repair Damaged Tissues

To obtain good relief and recovery you will need to repair some of your damaged tissues. There are several physical, medical, and nutritional measures you can do to promote repair of damaged tissue. Repair is the **ONLY** way to permanently reduce pain. Here are some recommended nutrition measures to promote repair of damaged tissues.

I. NUTRITIONAL SUPPLEMENTS

    a. Essential
   - i. Vitamin C, 2000 to 4000mg a day
   - ii. B_{12} 500 – 1000mcg a day
   - iii. Amino acid or collagen supplement

    b. Optional/best single amino acids
   - i. Carnitine
   - ii. Taurine

    c. Best minerals
   - i. Magnesium
   - ii. Boron
   - iii. Selenium

    d. Optional: Best single vitamins other than C and B_{12}
   - i. B_6
   - ii. D
   - iii. D_3

II. FOOD AND BEVERAGE INTAKE

    a. Your daily diet should consist of some protein, foods low in sugar and starch, and high in green vegetables

    b. Highly recommended: a protein food with each meal (seafood, meat, eggs, cottage cheese)

    c. Stop sugared drinks. Use low-sugar substitutes.

III. SUGAR AND CHOLESTEROL TESTING/TREATMENT: All persons with IP should have their sugar (glucose) and cholesterol tested. New research shows that excess glucose and cholesterol form "glycation" products that damage nerves and other tissues.

Appendix D. Difference Between Chronic and Intractable Pain

	IPS	CP
Pain is Constant (24/7)	Yes	No
Treatment is Daily (Around the Clock)	Yes	No
Elevated Blood Pressure and Pulse Rate	Yes	Seldom
Elevated Temperature and Breathing Rate	Yes	No
Anorexia/Malnutrition	Yes	No
Insomnia	Yes	No
Depression, Hopelessness	Yes	No
Endocrine Abnormalities (Hormones & Glucose)	Yes	No
Elevated Inflammatory Markers	Often	Seldom
Restriction of certain life activities (e.g. mobility)	Yes	Sometimes
Decreased capability for Requirements of Daily Living	Yes	No

Appendix E. Making the Most of Opioids

The oldest measure to make an opioid more effective has been to add a chemical agent that makes the opioid act "longer and stronger." This concept is known as "potentiation."

HISTORY: Various herbs or botanicals such as boswellia and cannabis were used with opium in ancient times. Physicians in the 1700's mixed alcohol with opium. British physicians combined aspirin with morphine around the turn of the 19th Century. Later they determined that a stimulant-type drug, including cocaine, made morphine more effective for the person with severe pain. This was called the Brompton Cocktail named after Brompton Hospital in London. After World War II, American pharmaceutical companies began combining the opioids codeine, hydrocodone, and oxycodone with aspirin, caffeine, acetaminophen, ibuprofen, and phenacetin. Today, the most popular potentiating combination is acetaminophen with codeine, hydrocodone (example: Vicodin®), and oxycodone (example: Percocet®).

MAIN MESSAGE

1. An opioid should almost NEVER be taken alone by a person with IP. Why? First, you don't get the full effect of the opioid. Second, without a potentiator, you will need to take a higher opioid dose when a lower one would suffice, so you will probably run out of opioids before you can obtain another prescription.

2. Every IP patient needs to identify at least two potentiators to take with your opioids.

SOME POTENTIATORS TO TRY:

Caffeine Tablet+	Adderall®
Mucuna+	Methylphenidate
Boswellia+	Dextroamphetamine
Gabapentin	Benadryl®+
Taurine+	GABA+
CBD Products+	

+=non-prescription

Appendix F. Sleep Medication for Intractable Pain

IP usually keeps one from getting enough sleep to attain maximal relief and recovery. Most persons with IP will need to take some medication to sleep. If your IP is mild, you may not need it.

SLEEP, RELIEF, AND RECOVERY
During sleep the brain replenishes biochemicals and hormones that provide pain control, memory, energy, endurance, motivation, reading and writing ability, and logical thinking.

SLEEP PATTERN

Most persons with IP must sleep in spurts of two to four hours. This is OK as long as you get six to eight hours of sleep time during each twenty-four-hour time period between 6:00 am to 6:00 am the next day.

TRADITIONAL PRESCRIPTION MEDICATIONS:

Restoril®, Ambien®, nortriptyline, gabapentin, Halcion®, amitriptyline, trazadone, Soma®

SLEEP BOOSTERS

Take a dose of your regular pain medication thirty to sixty minutes before bedtime. You can boost your regular sleep medication with non-prescription melatonin, tryptophan, glutamine, 5-HTP, Benadryl®, valerian root, or gamma amino butyric acid (GABA).

Appendix G. Best Remedies for Pain Flares

The standard treatment for severe pain flares has essentially remained the same for about a century: an injection or suppository of a short-acting opioid such as morphine, hydromorphone, or meperidine. About mid-way through the last century some short acting opioid suppositories were made-plain opium, morphine, or hydromorphone. In the last third of the last century sublingual or buccal (dissolve in the mouth) fentanyl was developed in the form of tablets, troches, oral spray, or lollipop.

Two non-opioid injections have been made in recent years for flare-up pain: ketorolac and ketamine.

ESSENTIAL FOR IP

Every person with IP must have a pre-set, strategy and plan for severe pain flares. Furthermore, the plan needs to be such that it can be done in your home-not at the emergency room or the hospital. Be prepared. Discuss your need for flare-up treatment with your medical practitioners.

MAJOR CAUSE OF OVER-DOSE

Many drug overdoses (OD's) happen when desperate patients don't have a potent short acting pain reliever at home and ready for emergency use. They try to self-treat an unexpected flare without a short-acting opioid.

Planning and preparation are the best prevention when you have IP. Have a plan in place for flares-ups.

SEE YOUR LOCAL DOCTOR AND PHARMACIST

Every IP patient needs to arrange with their local physician and pharmacist to have an emergency opioid injection or suppository for a severe flare. You need to be able to administer the injection or suppository at home, so you don't have to attend an emergency room.

Appendix H. How to Obtain Medical Help in Your Local Community

New opioid restrictions essentially mandate that persons who have IP should pursue physicians (MD) and nurse practitioners (NP) in their local community to provide necessary care.

FIRST REQUIREMENT: You must have a verifiable, anatomic diagnosis that is the cause of your IP. The fact that you have IP is not sufficient-you must know the cause of your IP.

Case Examples of What Not to Do:

> #1 A woman who was taking three different opioids suddenly found that her opioids quit providing pain relief. She consulted her local MD. When asked what caused her pain, neither she nor her husband knew her underlying cause of pain. They did not have an answer.

> #2 A woman on two opioids, wanted a letter from her physician to support her disability claim. When asked the cause of her pain, she didn't know, but her feet and legs hurt. Someone told her she might have fibromyalgia.

Note: Neither of the two cases here could produce a single page of medical records stating the cause of their pain. It is no wonder they couldn't locate a doctor to help.

HOW IS AN ANATOMIC DIAGNOSIS OBTAINED?

This requires a physical examination plus confirmation with an x-ray, MRI, photograph, blood test, electro conduction study, or biopsy. This information must be documented in your medical record. Equally important is to keep a copy of all test results in your personal possession-not in some doctor's office.

UNACCEPTABLE DIAGNOSES: The following are not usually considered specific enough diagnoses to obtain opioids or disability:

bad back, sciatica, failed back, sprain or strain, fibromyalgia, headache, accident, neck pain, fall

COMMON DIAGNOSES FOR IP

- Adhesive Arachnoiditis (AA)
- Herniated discs with complications
- Post-Stroke
- Reflex Sympathetic Dystrophy (RSD) or Chronic Regional Pain Syndrome (CRPS)
- Sickle Cell Disease
- Specific Arthritis (Psoriatic or other)
- Interstitial Cystitis
- Specific Neuropathy (familial, porphyria, diabetic, etc.)
- Traumatic Brain Injury (TBI)
- Genetic connective tissue/collagen disorders (Ehlers-Danlos Syndromes)

WHEN ASKED ABOUT YOUR NEED FOR CARE

Do NOT identify yourself as a "pain patient" in your attempt to secure a physician. Instead, state your specific disease diagnosis that causes pain. For example: I have (name your anatomic disease) which causes IP and other symptoms.

Appendix I: Opioid Substitutes and Potentiators

To cope with the new restrictions on opioids and benzodiazepines, all IP patients will have to quickly adjust. Here are some ideas to discuss with your family and medical practitioners.

AVAILABLE PRESCRIPTION OPIOIDS: Most local physicians can prescribe these two opioids:
1. Tramadol
2. Codeine-Tylenol®-combinations.

While "Better Than Nothing" you may have to build a pain control program with one, or both, of these two agents. You can do this with what is called potentiators and substitutes.

MAY BE AVAILABLE FROM LOCAL PRACTIONERS: If you have a set of hand-carry records which document the causes and complications of your IP, some medical practitioners will prescribe, local pharmacies will fill, and insurance companies will financially cover the following opioids:

1. Hydrocodone-acetaminophen (Vicodin®, Norco®) three-four a day
2. Oxycodone-acetaminophen (Percocet®) three-four a day
3. Plain oxycodone two-three a day

OPIOID SUBSTITUTES: These drugs have some opioid effect known in pharmacology as "opioid activity." They can be taken separately between opioid dosages, or they can be taken at the same time, to make your opioid "stronger" and last "longer."

NON-PRESCRIPTION
Kratom
Palmitoylethanolamide (PEA)
CBD/Marihuana
Taurine

PRESCRIPTION
Amphetamine Salts-(Adderall®)
Tizanidine
Methylphenidate (Ritalin®)
Clonidine

Ketamine
Oxytocin

Appendix J: Critical Necessity to Maintain Hormone Blood Levels

Some specific hormones are essential to find relief and recovery from IP. Why?

> #1. Opioid potency and effectiveness may decline and almost become useless if certain hormone blood levels drop below normal

> #2. Healing and repair of damaged tissue and suppression of inflammation simply can't happen if some hormones are too low.

CRITICAL HORMONES FOR TESTING: Cortisol, DHEA, Pregnenolone, Testosterone

Optional: Progesterone and estradiol

WHY DO HORMONES DROP

> √ Constant pain overstresses the body's hormone production system
> √ Opioids, benzodiazepines, and some other common pain-relieving drugs suppress hormone production.

HOW OFTEN TO TEST: Every four-six months

SYMPTOMS OF A LOW HORMONE LEVEL

Poor pain control
Fatigue/weakness

Loss of opioid effectiveness
Memory decline
Insomnia
Depression

WHAT IF MY DOCTOR WON'T ORDER A HORMONE TEST?

You don't need a doctor's order. One good source of laboratory testing is Life-Extension.
Contact: Life Extension: Phone- 1-800-678-8989,
Website: https://www.lifeextension.com/lab-testing

Appendix K: The Old-Fashioned Estrogen Shot

Not too many years ago a monthly estrogen shot was common in every community and given to post-menopausal women either in a doctor's office or taken at home. Women and physicians have become overly afraid of cancer due to estrogen. The fact is that the only estrogen cancer cases have been in women who took daily high doses of only certain, synthetic estrogen derivatives. There has not been a single reported case of cancer caused by a monthly injection of bioidentical estrogen.

OBSERVATIONS

An old-fashioned bioidentical estrogen injection given monthly may prevent and reduce pain. After menopause the production of estrogen shifts from the ovaries to the adrenal glands. If the adrenal glands are overly stressed from the constant pain, estrogen production can be greatly hampered. The addition of supplemental estrogen can greatly improve the healing of tissues and reduce pain.

THERAPEUTIC TRIAL

It is our belief that every non-menstruating female with IP should try a monthly, bioidentical estrogen injection. An alternative is oral bioidentical estrogen to be taken two-three days a week.

NATURAL HERBAL PRODUCTS

All women, pre-and post-menopausal, who have IP may benefit from a natural estrogenic herbal extract or blend of herbs. Herbs and plant derived hormonal agents that may be helpful are siberian rhubarb, chaste tree berries, dong quai, black cohosh, red clover, maca, shatavari. The hormonal precursor DHEA makes some estrogen and testosterone.

Appendix L: Tips to Reduce Descending Pain

Descending pain is electricity that is generated in the brain that travels downward from the head into muscles, nerves, fatty tissues, tendons, skin, and joints. Persons with IP, in contrast to simple, chronic pain, have what is called "descending pain." For good pain relief you will have to control descending pain.

TIPS TO CONTROL DESCENDING PAIN

1. DOPAMINE AND NORADRENALINE PRECURSORS: You can usually restore your natural levels of dopamine and noradrenaline with the amino acid precursors that make these neurotransmitters: phenylalanine or tyrosine. Take 1000 to 2000mg phenylalanine or tyrosine in the morning on an empty stomach. You can take them together or you can take one alone on alternate days. Take either phenylalanine or tyrosine at least five days per week. Take B_6 along with them for maximal effect.

2. DOPAMINE-NORADRENALINE SUBSITUTES: Take a dopamine-noradrenaline substitute in the morning as directed by your physician - amphetamine salts (Adderall®), phentermine, phendimetrazine, methylphenidate, dextroamphetamine, modafinil.

OPTIONAL: Take a descending pain blocker technically called an Alpha-2 receptor agonist: clonidine or tizanidine. These drugs may lose power and can become toxic. They are not usually as effective as actual dopamine-noradrenaline substitutes.

Appendix M: Low Dose Naltrexone - Choice for New IP Patients

A major advance in pain management is the discovery of low-dose naltrexone (LDN). It is now the preferred, first drug of choice for IP. LDN not only relieves pain but has anti-inflammatory and immune boosting properties on brain and spinal cord tissues.

WHO SHOULD TAKE LDN? Those persons who are not currently on daily opioids. A major purpose of LDN is to prevent the necessity of daily opioids.

PART OF A MULTI-DRUG PROGRAM: LDN should ideally be a part of a multi-drug program. A nerve conduction blocker (neuropathic) agent such as gabapentin or diazepam will almost always boost pain relief. A dopamine substitute such as Adderall®, or Ritalin®, is very helpful. Routinely recommended are standard anti-inflammatory (e.g., Ketorolac) and tissue healing (anabolic) agents (e.g., DHEA). A pain flare medication should also be handy and ready. Some patients taking LDN can occasionally take a low dose of tramadol, codeine, or hydrocodone for pain flares. Other flare medications include ketamine, CBD, medical marijuana, ibuprofen(800mg.) oxytocin, kratom, and ketorolac.

*CAUTION AND WARNING: Persons who currently take daily opioids must withdraw from daily opioids before starting LDN. In our studies patients sometimes became "deathly" ill if they took LDN while still on opioids. Severe withdrawal may set in, pain relief will diminish, and, at worst, a cardiac-adrenal crisis may be precipitated.

DOSAGE: Starting dosage is usually 0.5 – 1.0 milligram(mg.) taken twice a day. The average maintenance dose is about 3.0 – 5.0mg. taken twice a day. The maximum is about 7.0mg. taken twice a day.

STAY WITH WHAT IS WORKING: If one has IP and is currently on a regimen including opioids that satisfactorily reduces pain, there is no medical reason to switch to LDN.

HISTORICAL PHOTOGRAPHS

There is a magnificent and caring history surrounding treatment of intractable pain patients. While the name "intractable" may not have been used, historical descriptions of persons with this type of pain make it clear that they had constant, incurable pain. This is the basic definition of "intractable."

I've created a pictorial history of intractable pain treatment beginning with Dr. John Fothergill. He was the esteemed British physician in the 1700's who tackled the intractable pain of incurable, terminal tuberculosis with a concoction of opium and alcohol. My rendition of these events ends when I started the first public health facility in 1975, to treat both persons who were addicted to the opioid, heroin, and those who had intractable pain.

Two very important precepts historically stand out. Some caring and diligent physicians believed that no one should have to suffer or die in intractable pain. The other precept is that life should not be shortened by depriving any intractable pain patient of opioids or other pain-relieving drugs. It has been well-known among physicians over the past two centuries that severe, untreated pain shortens life.

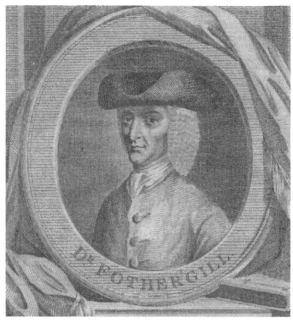

John Fothergill (1712-1780)

John Fothergill was the preeminent physician in London during the 1700's. He was the first to recognize and publish that pain could best be treated with a combination of opium and alcohol. His formula for the pain, cough, and depression of incurable, fatal tuberculosis (called "consumption") was "one-half ounce of pure white opium seeds in a pint of Bristol." This concoction established the scientific principle that opioids should be combined with a "potentiator" for maximum effect. Opium and alcohol combinations were used for war wounds by the physicians under the command of George Washington in the Revolutionary War.

Reference

Wilber CK. Revolutionary Medicine, Globe Pequot Press. Guilford, Connecticut. 1980

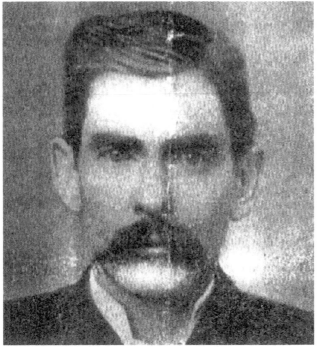

John Henry "Doc" Holliday (1851-1887)

In the 1800's "Doc" Holliday was a dentist who became famous as a gunfighter in Dodge City, Kansas and Tombstone, Arizona including the "shoot-out" at the OK Corral. He had a lung disease believed to be tuberculosis or a related disease, and he used a combination of opium and alcohol for pain relief. Because of his medical knowledge of medicines, he was probably able to live much longer than would have been expected for a person with his condition.

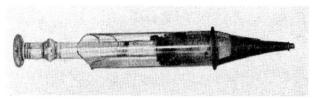

DR. WOOD'S ORIGINAL SYRINGE

A major advance in the treatment of intractable pain was the development of a syringe that could inject morphine. Although various injection syringes were initially made, it was the Scottish physician Alexander Wood, who in 1853, first combined a hallow steel needle with a proper syringe that could inject morphine into a human. Pictured here is Dr. Wood's original syringe.

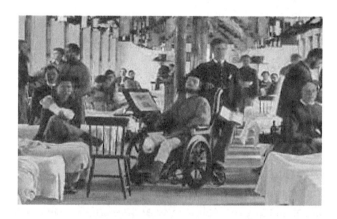

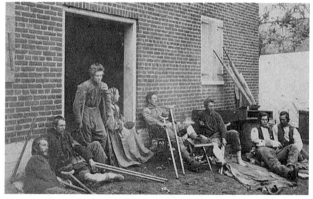

INJURED CIVIL WAR VETERANS

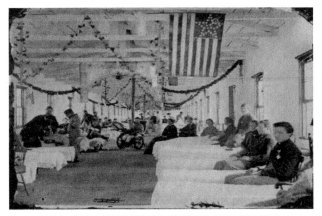

CIVIL WAR SOLDIERS RECEIVING TREATMENT

The first concerted attempt to treat intractable pain in the United States was to relieve the pain caused by neurologic injuries incurred by soldiers in the Civil War. Soldiers particularly developed severe pain in their arms, legs, and feet. This pain was called "causalgia." Today it is known as reflex sympathetic dystrophy (RSD), or complex regional pain syndrome (CRPS). Morphine was given to injured soldiers, in many cases, for several years after the war.

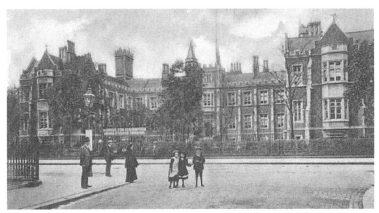

Royal Brompton Hospital - Circa 1890

In 1896, physicians at the Brompton Hospital in London, England began treating severe intractable pain. They discovered that opioids should be mixed with stimulants for maximal effect. Their original mixture contained morphine and cocaine. Later it was called the "Brompton Cocktail." The Brompton Hospital formulary in 1957 listed these ingredients:

Morphine hydrochloride, ¼ grain (15mg)
Cocaine hydrochloride, 1/6 grain (10mg)
Alcohol 90% (2ml)
Syrup,4ml
Chloroform water ½ fl. (15ml)

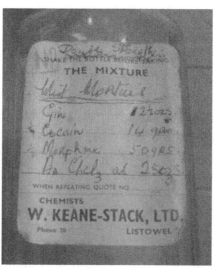

An Original Prescription for the Brompton Cocktail

Federal Medical Center, Lexington

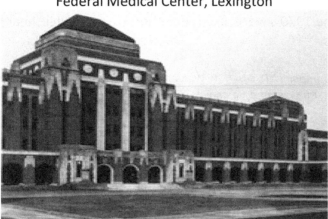

THE NARCOTIC FARM

The site opened on May 15, 1935 on 1,000 acres under the name "United States Narcotic Farm." The name was later changed to the "U.S. Public Health Service Hospital." In 1967, it changed its name again to "National Institute of Mental Health, Clinical Research Center." Its original purpose was to treat people who voluntarily were admitted with drug abuse problems and treat them, with mostly experimental treatments. It was the first of its kind in the United States. The site included a farm where patients would work. Although initially opened for volunteers, it later became a facility where addict-prisoners were sent. In 1974 the "farm" was closed as a therapeutic center for drug addicts, and in 1990 it was declared a Federal Medical Center for seriously ill Federal prisoners. Prior to 1976, within the hospital was a research unit to find addiction treatments as well as non-addicting pain treatment drugs. After World War II, narcotic formulas were taken from the Germans and tested at the center. Part of the testing was administration of the test drugs to hospitalized addicts. This research program developed methadone and other opioid-related compounds which are currently used today. Physicians who staffed the hospital were public health physicians and established the notion that addiction and intractable pain should be treated by such physicians. Consequently, physicians who started addiction and intractable pain treatment in America's cities in the 1970's were, like the author, trained public health physicians.

Reference: Campbell ND, Olsen JP, Walden L. The Narcotic Farm: the rise and fall of America's first prison for drug addicts. Harry Abrams New York, NY 2008.

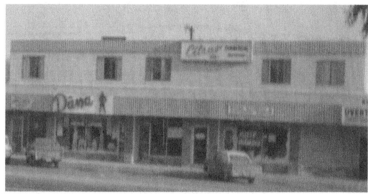

Author's Public Health Facility for Addiction and Intractable Pain – Circa 1980

The Public Health Facility in West Covina, California (East of Downtown Los Angeles) was established in 1975. The clinic was upstairs over a row of commercial establishments. The center was initially located and financed through the Los Angeles County Public Health Foundation. It was directed by the author who had just obtained his doctorate in public health. The facility provided standard public health services for tuberculosis, sexually transmitted diseases, vaccinations, family planning, and well-baby care. A methadone clinic for heroin addicts was started as well as an intractable pain program. The first intractable pain patients were either referred from the regional cancer hospital (City of Hope) or were desperate, non-addict intractable pain patients who had heard that methadone had become available to treat their pain.

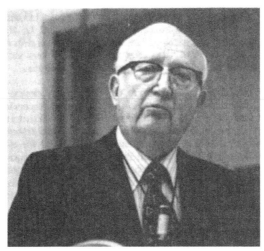

Frank Fraser, MD

Dr. Fraser became a research physician in 1949 at the Federal Narcotic Facility in Lexington, Kentucky. He developed methodologies to test and determine the addiction and pain relief potential of many compounds. Testing included administration of drugs to inmates. A major discovery by Dr. Fraser were drugs that are technically called mixed agonist-antagonist compounds which provide good pain relief with limited addiction potential. His methods led to the development of pentazocine and today's buprenorphine. After 1963 he became a research consultant for Eli Lilly and the Federal research agencies concerned with addiction and pain relief. When the author began to develop the Nation's first community-based public health addiction and intractable pain outpatient facility in 1975, Dr. Fraser was sent by his sponsors to West Covina, CA on several occasions to consult with and train the author. At that time, Dr. Fraser possessed more knowledge of addiction and pain than any other physician in the United States, and he believed that only physicians who understood the difference between opioid addiction and intractable pain should attempt long-term treatment with narcotics.

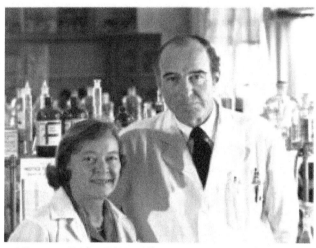

Vincent Dole, MD and Marie Nyswander, MD

Vincent Dole (1913-2006) along with his wife, Marie Nyswander (1919 –1986) , were the physicians who developed the use of methadone to treat heroin addiction. Both were originally research physicians at the Federal Narcotic Facility in Lexington, Kentucky. They were recruited away to New York in the early 1960's by the Rockefeller Foundation to find a treatment for heroin addiction which was plaguing New York and other metropolitan areas. The author became aware of their work and administered methadone to addicted US Army soldiers when he served as a US Army Medical Officer in Germany in the late 1960's. Although these physicians are best known for their addiction efforts, they also established how intractable pain should be treated. They both shared the belief that heroin and other opioid addictions had a genetic, irreversible make-up that often-required methadone to suppress their craving for opioids. Drs. Dole and Nyswander believed that intractable pain should be treated with a low, daily dose of methadone since it was long-acting. Pain flares or what they called "breakthrough" pain were treated with a short-acting opioid. This procedure was primarily used for intractable pain until the commercial development of the fentanyl patch and long-acting oxycodone (Oxycontin®) which were initially (and many believe falsely) promoted for superior intractable pain treatment compared to the "methadone/short-acting opioid" protocol. It is noteworthy that Dr. Dole received the distinguished 1988 Albert Lasker Award for Clinical Medical Research.

In 1972, when the author was transferred from the US Army Medical Corp to the United States Public Health Service as an Academic Fellow, he spent time training with Dole and Nyswander at Rockefeller Center to learn their methods of treating both opioid addiction and intractable pain. It was the general belief of Dole and Nyswander, in the 1970's and 80's, that public health physicians should be the primary physicians to use opioids in the treatment of both addiction and intractable pain.

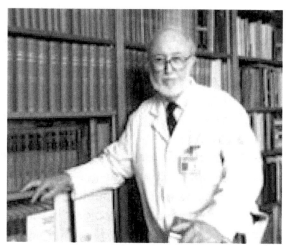

Raymond W. Houde, MD

Dr. Houde was a physician who specialized in treating cancer pain. While at Sloan-Kettering Hospital in New York, he developed the concept of morphine equivalence. His table of morphine potency was to assist physicians when they needed to change opioids. The concept of morphine potency or equivalence has recently been adopted to regulate and restrict opioid use which was never even considered or intended by Dr. Houde. It was strictly a clinical tool. The author was mentored by Dr. Houde in the first years of his intractable pain clinic as the focus was greatly on treating late-stage or post-cancer patients. These patients often suffered pain from tissue destruction of the cancer and surrounding tissue by mutilating surgery, or radiation. Dr. Houde believed that opioid dosages should be titrated upward, over time, regardless of dosage to ensure pain relief and allow the patient to maintain mental and physical function. He firmly believed that no one should die in pain or that life should be shortened by deprivation of opioids.

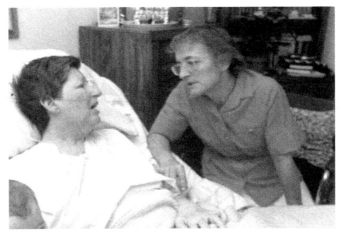

Elisabeth Kubler Ross

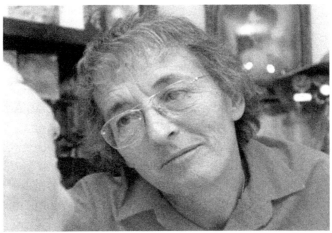

Elisabeth Kübler-Ross, M.D. (1926 – 2004)

Dr. Ross championed end-of-life care and admonished other physicians to have open and honest conversations with patients about death and dying. The author started his original clinic in 1975, in part, to emulate Dr. Kubler Ross in the care of end-of-life patients. He surprisingly found that some end-of-life patients with intractable pain could prolong their life by months or years if they were treated with a combination of opioids and stimulant drugs.

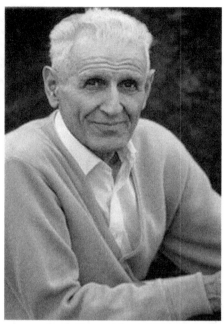

Jack Kevorkian, M.D.

Dr. Murad Jacob "Jack" Kevorkian (1928 – 2011) was an American pathologist and euthanasia proponent. He publicly championed a terminal patient's right to die by physician-assisted suicide, embodied in his quote, "Dying is not a crime." He was the first and most famous physician to advocate and practice assisted suicide. Dr. Kevorkian contacted the author and said he had patients who didn't wish to die if they could only get intractable pain care. Consequently, some referrals were accepted by the author from Dr. Kevorkian, and they lived for several more years with intractable pain care.

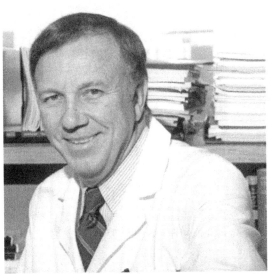

Dr. C. Stratton Hill, Jr., M.D. (1928-2015)

Dr. Hill was the Texas physician who sponsored and lobbied the Texas Legislature to pass the first intractable pain law in 1990. The intent of the law was to allow physicians to prescribe opioids to bonafide, intractable pain patients without fear of prosecution by State Medical Boards and Departments of Justice. Intractable pain was defined as "incurable by any known means." Dr. Hill had been a president of the Texas Medical Association and was an expert in treating cancer and other causes of intractable pain. He obtained the definition of intractable pain and criteria for the necessity of opioids from the work and publications of the former work of the British Intractable Pain Society.

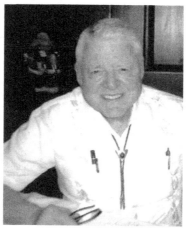

Harvey Rose MD 1932-2008

Shortly after Texas passed their Intractable Pain Act in 1990, Dr. Rose and State Senator Leroy Greene lobbied the California Legislature and Governor to pass an Intractable Pain Act that was essentially identical to the Texas Act. Along with the author, Dr. Rose and Senator Greene later convinced the California Legislature to enact the California Pain Patients' Bill of Rights in 1998. These legislative achievements fostered a significant movement of research and treatment of intractable pain for the following twenty years.

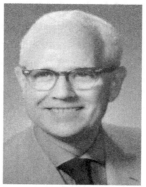

State Senator Leroy F. Greene (1918 – 2002)

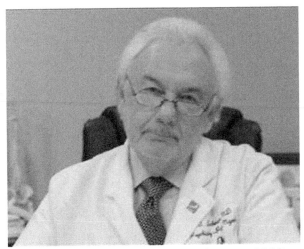

Dr. Joel Frederick Simon Hochman - 2010

In 1972 the author was transferred from the United States Army Medical Corp to the United States Public Health Service and assigned to the UCLA School of Public Health as an Academic Fellow. At that time, he met Dr. Hochman who was a psychiatric resident. Both of us immediately became friends and colleagues as we believed that addiction, alcoholism, and intractable pain were emerging as dominant public health issues. This mutual belief led our colleagues to brand us as "misguided mavericks." Dr. Hochman went on to become an expert in intractable pain management, leading him to establish the National Foundation for the Treatment of Pain in 1998. As a tireless and powerful advocate for the rights of others to be free from needless suffering, he fought and won many regulatory battles on their behalf at times under grave pressure and unrelenting adversity. Clinically, he believed that opioid dosages should be titrated upward over time to a point that pain was relieved and biologic functions were retained so the patient would have a good quality of life.

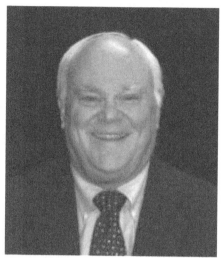

Dr. Jeffery Reinking 1945 – 2011

Dr. Reinking and the author partnered to establish intractable pain clinics in Northern California between 1998 and 2010. He was a most gregarious and lovable man who was a professional member of a number of national and international organizations including the International Association for the Study of Pain, the American Academy of Pain Medicine, the International Association of Pain and Chemical Dependency and the American Medical Association. Dr. Reinking was recognized as a pioneer in the interdisciplinary approach to the treatment of chronic pain. In his work he realized that a sub-group of chronic pain patients had constant, intractable pain that required on-going medical treatment. At the time of his death, he had about two dozen intractable pain patients who had taken high, daily dosages of opioids for twenty to thirty years. The author evaluated these patients and found they functioned well mentally and physically. Minor endocrine (hormonal) deficiencies were the only physiologic abnormalities found in Dr. Reinking's patients. The author best remembers Dr. Reinking making this statement, "I can't explain it, but the intractable pain patients who take a lot of vitamins and supplements just do a lot better."

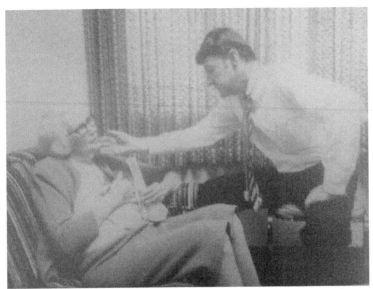

Author with Cancer Patient – Circa 1980

This patient had most of her face removed due to cancer of her facial bones. She self-administered methadone or morphine through an implanted tube into her stomach. Fortunately, cancer treatment with chemotherapy and radiation in the past forty years has progressively improved to the point that mutilating surgery and intractable pain care are no longer needed in the majority of cases. This picture originally appeared in National Geographic Magazine as part of a story on opium.

INDEX

2021 Reprint of the Original

Published as a public service by the Tennant Foundation.
Medical Research and Education Projects
Tennant Foundation
336-338 S. Glendora Ave.
West Covina, CA 91790
626-716-2689
Fax: 626-919-7497
E-mail: tennantfoundation92@gmail.com
Websites: www.arachnoiditishope.com
www.intractablepainsyndrome.com

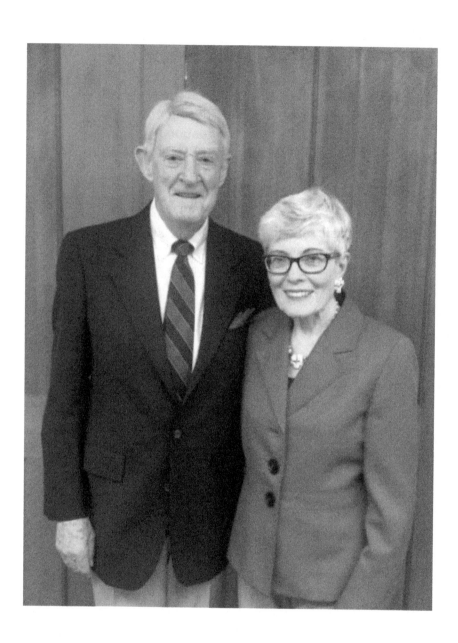

About The Author

Forest Tennant has spent most of his medical career as a practicing physician and researcher in the fields of addiction and pain medicine. He has published over 300 scientific articles and books in these fields. For his efforts he was recently given a "50 Year Achievement" award by "Pain Week." In this 50-year span he has been a US Army Medical Officer, UCLA Professor, Public Health Physician, Drug Advisor for the Los Angeles Dodgers, NASCAR, and the National Football League. He was editor of Practical Pain Management for 12 years. He recently retired from clinical practice to do research on intractable pain and the spinal cord disorder known as arachnoiditis. He and his wife, Miriam, have been married 55 years and they split their residence between West Covina, California and Wichita, Kansas, where they headquarter their real-estate company, Tennant Homes. Their charitable giving and medical research are sponsored by the Tennant Foundation.

Other Books by Forest Tennant

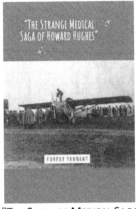

"THE STRANGE MEDICAL SAGA
OF HOWARD HUGHES"
ISBN: 9781955934091
LOC: 2021912855

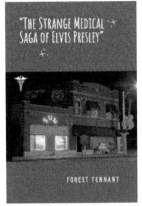

"THE STRANGE MEDICAL SAGA
OF ELVIS PRESLEY"
ISBN: 9781955934008
LOC: 2021911718

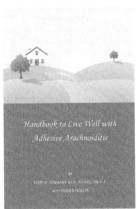

"HANDBOOK TO LIVE WELL WITH ADHESIVE
ARACHNOIDITIS"
ISBN: 978195934060
LOC: 2021912718

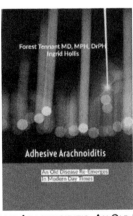

"ADHESIVE ARACHNOIDITIS: AN OLD DISEASE
RE-EMERGES IN MODERN TIMES"
ISBN: 9781955934039
LOC:2021912467

Available on Amazon and where books are sold

Made in the USA
Middletown, DE
22 June 2023

33227416R00070